Sugar Surfing: Changing Lives

Here's what people are already saying about *Sugar Surfing*™:

"Successful type 1 diabetes management requires a dynamic thought process. Sugar Surfing lays this out in a way such that anyone can improve their management skills. What gets measured and analyzed gets improved." - Jon & Robbie Kizer, Tannum Sands, QLD, Australia (son Joshua with type 1 diabetes since 2010)

"Matthew has now been taught to use his Sugar Surfing skills at school to bolus when he sees a rise in his blood sugar. He also eats small amounts when he starts to see a drop. He is doing his best to not drop too low that he needs to go to the clinic, or to allow his blood sugar to get too high in that it means having to repeat school work. Sugar Surfing has been an incredibly positive learning & teaching method for our family." - The Boardman family, Houston, Texas (son Matthew with type 1 diabetes since 2012)

"I am very excited that Dr. Ponder has put his perspective toward managing T1D into a concise and well-written book that we can share with others." - Mike Barry, Chicago Illinois (type 1 diabetes since 1984)

"With what I learned from Sugar Surfing I soon found the confidence to experiment in ways that I'd not even dreamt about before; micro-bolusing to nudge the levels down is one of my favourites! I now feel empowered to surf. I've not had a single severe hypo since I began using Dr. Ponder's lessons and hope I'll never darken the doors of another emergency department with a diabetes related problem. Such visits are totally avoidable if you are committed to becoming a Sugar Surfer and take appropriate precautions." - Lis Warren, London United Kingdom (type 1 diabetes since 1965)

"By using the principles of Sugar Surfing I was able to lower my A1C from 7.4 to 6.3 and then to 6.0. Having a lower A1C makes me happy, no doubt there, and using Sugar Surfing techniques empowers me with this disease. I know that I can manage it, make decisions in the moment, and get desired results. Sugar Surfing allows me to be proactive; not to wait for someone to tell me what I should have done days or months ago." - BettyAnn Foster, Alpine Texas (Latent Autoimmune Diabetes of Adults (LADA) since 2011)

"Armed with the empowering philosophy of Sugar Surfing, you know how to read the BG curves and the patterns, how to respond without over-responding and how to deal with just about any situation that comes up. The days now flow with a more flexible and "normal" rhythm. Best of all, I know I'm not alone no matter what the day's challenges." - Marcy and Robert Garriott, Austin, Texas (Grand Aunt and Uncle of 6 year old with type 1 diabetes)

"How do you teach people to go against accepted principles and do it safely? ...YOU TEACH SUGAR SURFING!!! Thank you Stephen and Kevin for bringing to us all this amazing combination of good science, common sense and the individual power of self-reliance. This new method makes it practical to win with CGM!!!" - Della Matheson RN, CDE, Miami Florida (Diabetes Research Nurse, T1D for 33 years)

"Sugar Surfing is freedom. Knowing that effective management requires more than just reacting to a number in time allows enormous flexibility in controlling diabetes. Freedom to learn, predict and ultimately master diabetes management." - Whit Talbot, Houston, Texas (type 1 diabetes since 1990)

"As a d-mom, I love Sugar Surfing the most overnight. My 10 year old daughter Savannah has always had hugely variable BGs and insulin needs overnight. Sugar Surfing has let us see and respond to what's going on much sooner. That means 'high' nights are now 250 instead of 400. Surfing gives us more tools in our toolbox, helps us gain knowledge and use it in the most effective way possible." - Angela Richard, Houston, Texas

"I am passionate that more children and adults with T1D benefit from Dr Ponder's knowledge and skills as we have. Plus, I'm optimistic that 'Sugar Surfing' (the book) can help to achieve that end. Please keep up the amazing work!" - Elle Dormer, London United Kingdom, (mum to Indy Dormer 4yrs old; diagnosed at 2.5 yrs)

"Sugar Surfing has given us a whole new outlook on diabetes management for our daughter. We strive as a family to maintain an excellent level of control while still allowing our child to be a child. Sugar Surfing inspires us to 'ride the waves' and to always keep moving forward and to keep trying. Learning to micro-carb and to give insulin 'nudges' are fantastic tools. Our A1C proves that it works. Thank you Dr. Ponder, truly, for everything." - The Vieau Family. Ottawa, ON, Canada. (Daughter Devyn diagnosed with type 1 diabetes in 2012)

"We are so happy since we began to Sugar Surf. It was the turning of the tide; a life changer. We have been Sugar Surfing ever since. It takes patience, perseverance, the ability to learn from failures and a commitment to being all you can be! The basics were AMAZING. With every success we high-fived and felt like one of those inspirational posters… WE COULD EAT ANYTHING!!! - Daniel & Jamie O'Flaherty, Denton, Texas (parents of Shannon age 13, T1D kid, Sugar Surfer)

"Sugar surfing is not just something a person does. It is an ever-changing way of life. It opened my eyes to how lack of sleep, stress, activity, food and not eating affect my glucose levels. It makes me a better doctor, husband, sibling and son while maintaining a sub-six A1C! As I've learned from Dr. Ponder and Kevin in the past, if a person is looking for a cure for diabetes – a way in which one can live as if diabetes did not exist – this is it." - Blake Nichols MD, Dallas, Texas (type 1 diabetes for 25 years, Sugar Surfing over one and a half years).

"To me Sugar Surfing is the absolute BEST name for what we do. And, when I think of that term 'surfing' in relation to diabetes I think of us riding the top of the wave; BG's in range and the ideal place to be. When his numbers start to go high or low is when we fall off the wave so making little corrections along the way keeps us on top of the wave. It's ALL a balancing act. It's a science really because there are so many factors; insulin, food, exercise, stress, etc... Dr. Ponder has taught me SO much about this concept. I am amazed by him & truly grateful to him every day for saving my son & teaching me how to help him thrive with these incredible tools & concepts." - Jennifer Urias, Midland, Texas (son Quintin now 8 years old; diagnosed Nov 17, 2011 at age 5).

The publisher takes no responsibility for the use of any of the materials or methods described in this book, nor for the products thereof. The name "mediself press" is a trademark of Type1 Technology Ventures, LLC. Printed in the United States of America.

ISBN	978 – 9962539 – 0 – 1
Font:	Palatino, 10pt.
Editor:	Patricia Ponder
Original Art:	Jackson Ponder
Cover Design:	Alexis Agoustari
Photography:	Stephen Ponder and Kevin McMahon

Questions regarding ordering and the content of this book should be addressed to **http://sugarsurfing.com**

Proceeds from the sale of this book are used to help fund Stephen Ponder's Sugar Surfing workshops and education programs.

SUGAR SURFING™

Sugar Surfing

How to manage type 1 diabetes in a modern world.

Stephen W. Ponder MD, FAAP, CDE

Kevin L. McMahon

Foreword

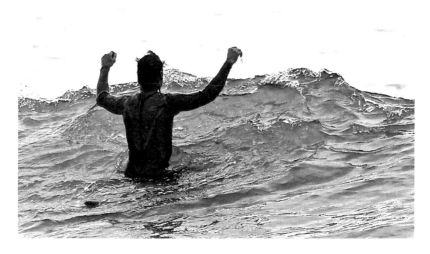

Sugar Surfing is truly a magical book in many ways. It is an account of a man's very long journey with type 1 diabetes. It is not only from the perspective of a down to earth hard working individual wanting to overcome and conquer the challenges of living with type 1 diabetes in the dark ages, but also from the view point of an incredible pediatric endocrinologist (diabetes specialist) who has devoted his career to taking care of others and teaching the future generation of doctors how to take better care of people with diabetes.

One of the greatest challenges for you as a person with diabetes is to become your own advocate and be knowledgeable about your condition so that you can obtain the best care possible. Sugar Surfing not only motivates you, but also explains the complexities of diabetes in a way that I have never experienced before. The facts of this complicated and multifaceted condition are explained in a way that is not only easy to understand, but also extremely interesting, which keeps you wanting to read more.

Sugar Surfing reaches out to the young and the old living with diabetes and just as important to the family members and loved ones who are helping to support someone with diabetes. Of the many books about diabetes, "Sugar Surfing" talks to the entire diabetes village… even to health care professionals interested in this area of medicine and to those already in the field of diabetes. Education is the key and I do not think there is a more effective communicator and motivator than Stephen Ponder.

There is contagiousness to Sugar Surfing because it reads like a novel. I say novel because once again it feels like an epic story of Dr. Ponder's journey from childhood diabetes to the modern era... teaching us along the way!

Sugar Surfing is truly a unique experience.

- Steve Edelman, MD

Dr. Edelman has strong interests in education and patient advocacy. He is the founder and director of Taking Control of Your Diabetes (TCOYD - http://tcoyd.org), a not-for-profit organization with the goal of teaching and motivating patients in diabetes self-care. Since 1995, TCOYD has reached hundreds of thousands of people living with diabetes through a variety of education portals including national conferences, publications, television, and community programs.

Preface

Compared to today, diabetes care in the 1960's seems medieval. But there is one element of daily diabetes care then that is still with us today; the concept of static thinking. For decades, my care was pre-set and rigidly prescribed: the food (what I could and couldn't eat) and the insulin (the same dose each day, often for years). Results of my urine tests didn't change anything until at least a doctor visit occurred and even then my prescriptions might have remained the same.

A "lance" (small disposable metal blade) was used to gouge my thumb (more ouch!) and milk out enough blood into a tube to send to the lab on the morning of a doctor visit. This was the way my diabetes control was judged: with a single blood sugar sample. Hemoglobin A1C tests were still years away. Yet in spite of all this I largely lived life like anyone else. I had the same minor illnesses, injuries, and life's ups and downs as any other child, but my daily diabetes care regimen was largely written in stone.

Through my own personal journey of trial and error I ultimately learned that I could improve my overall sense of well-being, not just my blood sugar control, by managing my diabetes "in the moment". Thanks to the development of the current generation of continuous glucose monitoring sensors it's now possible and practical to take a dynamic approach to self-care. I aim to share my journey of discovery with others.

This book is the culmination of my half century of living with type 1 diabetes; my wins and my losses. My hope is that by sharing my experiences, this book will help others who are ready to shift their diabetes care mindset from the mostly static approach I was trapped in for years. The pages that follow share my discoveries of something much more flexible; what I like to call dynamic diabetes management... but it's more fun to call it 'Sugar Surfing'.

This book is for anyone with diabetes who uses insulin therapy, but it has greatest relevance to those with type 1 diabetes or their loved ones who help them in its day to day management. Notice that I didn't say insulin pump therapy. Whether you pump or inject, this book is for you. Although this book might seem aimed at an experienced person with diabetes, I think it is well suited for the newly diagnosed individuals and families as well. Dynamic diabetes management is the future. While some persons may not ever be able to shift from the static, prescriptive approach to care, I feel there are many persons with type 1 diabetes who have been looking for a better way, an empowering approach, and have not yet found it. Sugar Surfing is what you might be looking for but I'll let you be the judge.

I will share with you how to coach yourself into better diabetes control. My method is based on a fundamental principle of how I manage myself as well as how I educate and support patients and families with diabetes. The guiding principle is that I (the doctor) don't "manage" my patient's diabetes. I never could and I never will. The reason is straightforward. I can't make all the hundreds of decisions and choices needed to manage a patient's blood sugar from one moment to the next.

I strongly recommend you master the basic principles of Sugar Surfing before attempting any of the advanced methods found in the chapters toward the end. Experienced surfers first master the small waves on a well maintained and balanced surfboard before ever attempting any sophisticated maneuvers.

Likewise, experienced Sugar Surfers must learn and practice basic skills each day if the advanced methods described later in the book are ever to be safely attempted and of benefit. You might only rarely use the advanced techniques. I've included many annotated examples to describe important concepts or techniques. Refer to them often as you tackle a new skill. When I meet you at one of my workshops I hope to see a worn out and battered copy of Sugar Surfing!

Much of what is written about in the first sections of the book should be practiced each and every day. Good ocean surfing technique starts with appropriate board selection, stance and balance. As you progress, a solid understanding of how waves shift, drift and roll become paramount to improving your skills in search of "The Perfect Wave". Sugar Surfers know how to maintain a well calibrated Continuous Glucose Monitoring (CGM) device, arrive at and maintain the right basal insulin delivery (through injection or insulin pump), properly assess the time required for insulin and food to exert effects on blood sugar levels, and master the art of micro-dosing insulin and micro-carbing food. The parallels are uncanny.

Expert surfers fall off their boards, wipeout and have off days, too. This book is not about how to achieve perfection. It's about how to learn from failure, break through barriers often placed by others and ourselves, learn to individualize our diabetes care, build self-confidence, figure out how to keep our heads above water and perhaps most of all, stay engaged. The surfer who ignores the ocean won't be enjoying their day for long. In other words, manage in the moment. But more importantly "enjoy the ride".

This book would have been impossible without the help of several people who are very close to me. My wife Patsy helped out at a critical moment to become our senior editor for which I am forever grateful while my talented son Jackson contributed several unique illustrations including the cover art. My good friend and co-author, Kevin McMahon, not only encouraged me to write this book but also helped me to find my voice. We've worked closely over the past 13 years on numerous projects aimed at improving the lives of children, teens and adults with diabetes and their families. Like me, Kevin's life was irrevocably changed when the younger of his two daughter's was diagnosed with type 1 diabetes at age two.

Let's start surfing!

Pro Surfers Need Sponsors

This first edition of Sugar Surfing has been supported by a unique 21st century grassroots mechanism: crowdsourcing. More than 400 people stepped up to make this book happen and you can read some of their names and dedications at the bottom of most pages of this book.

Over 25 years ago while working on staff at the Texas Lions Camp for Children with Diabetes, I befriended someone with whom I would maintain a lifelong personal and professional relationship in all matters diabetes; Gwen Gerlofs. Like me, Gwen had dedicated her life to improving the lives of others with diabetes through working and innovating from within the emerging diabetes pharmaceutical and technology industry of the 1990's. Not long after we began our friendship, she founded PumpsIt, Inc. which has grown to be a major national distributor of advanced diabetes technologies and education. Gwen continues in her role as CEO of that Houston, Texas based company today.

I want to dedicate this page to Gwen and her excellent team at PumpsIt, Inc. (http://pumpsit.com) for coming on board as our Industry Sponsor. Her support means we get to help create more Sugar Surfers by reaching into the hearts and minds of even more people with type 1 diabetes and those who care for them.

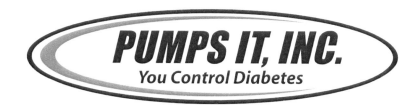

Contents

Disclaimer

Sugar Surfing is a process, not a result. Managing your diabetes in the moment aided by information provided by a real time CGM relies on more than just your personal bank of diabetes self-care knowledge. Ultimately, your success will require patience, personal consistency, and a good dose of resiliency. As with any special skill or ability you've mastered, commitment and dedication are needed to develop your basic competencies first. Full proficiency and expertise will follow. As the famous saying goes: "Rome wasn't built in a day".

I also wish to make sure the reader understands that anyone seeking to develop their own Sugar Surfing skills is first advised to consult about this with their own diabetes care provider. The materials in this book are not intended to represent a prescribed course of medical action or therapy for any individual or group. It's certainly not intended to replace the medical care, education and training received from a licensed health care professional. The overall purpose of this book is to enhance the reader's overall understanding and comprehension of their diabetes and its management.

Any new or cutting edge approach will have its detractors. Sugar Surfing is no different. While many of the tools described in this book are based on well established diabetes self-care principles, some may not be recommended or embraced by your diabetes care provider. Use of some of these surfing tools might be felt to be ill-advised based on your unique situation, age, or life circumstances.

In some cases, your health care provider might not be aware that Sugar Surfing even exists. That's the downside of a new paradigm. Therefore "no" might be the first answer you hear. As a physician, I understand and respect this conservative approach. This is why I also spend my time educating providers regarding Sugar Surfing as an option for diabetes care. Embracing new methods takes time and this book is part of my strategy for change.

I figure that as more persons inquire about Sugar Surfing with their doctors or share examples of their success using these tools, it will begin to change hearts and minds of some doctors and diabetes educators. Nevertheless, some of you might be met with a flat-out ban on a particular Sugar Surfing 'move' I might discuss. To be helpful, whenever controversy is likely, I will discuss its pros and cons in the event that you need to debate it with your diabetes provider.

Positive or negative outcomes which result from one's own diabetes self-care choices are the consequences of the actions of the individual, not the content of this book. Whenever tighter control of your diabetes is the goal, there is an increased risk for adverse events, including extremes of blood sugar, changes in weight, or in very rare cases disability or even death. With diabetes, as with life in general, risk is always present. Learning to manage risk well is part of quality diabetes self-care. I prefer to think of Sugar Surfing as a path to improved understanding, control and personal "ownership" of one's diabetes, but any discipline can be misused or applied improperly.

We stray from the path, all of us, from time to time. That doesn't make us bad, it makes us human. I'm no different. There are days when I am far more careful and meticulous than others. There are some days when I'm very attentive to what and how much I eat. But I too have days when I want to eat anything and everything, lay around, do nothing and skip meals. I must say I still keep an eye on my sensor tracings and apply what I've learned to buffer the impact on my blood sugar/blood glucose (BG) tracings. Guess what? I have roller coaster days just like everyone else.

I'm confident that if you follow these guidelines, be safe and apply them to your own situation, you can break through those barriers which may be holding you back.

Finally, machines break. Machines used to manage diabetes are designed with a level of inaccuracy built-in. The Sugar Surfing method is built upon frequent feedback from CGM devices and BG meters. We must always be wary and diligent when considering the data and information displayed by them. Always consider the data from these devices with the many caveats described in your specific device manufacturer's user guide.

Taking action on the wrong data and information can result in seriously catastrophic results. Always practice safe surfing.

Sugar Surfing for Kids

Much of the material in this book might be considered strictly for adults; empowered adults at that. But the principles of Sugar Surfing apply to persons with diabetes of all ages. I know families of toddlers, pre-teens and teens who apply these concepts in their daily approach to diabetes care. Of course all the same basic concepts apply: proper sensor calibration, basal confidence, timing, micro-dosing and micro-carbing.

This book contains a chapter specific to Sugar Surfing as it applies to children and teens. While the main concepts are the same, the chapter provides tips for engaging your child or teen in self-care as well as practical tips for 'Jr. Sugar Surfers' or kids who want to learn how to Surf.

Introduction

Why am I writing a book you ask? Kevin McMahon and I were talking sports analogies and the idea of creating a diabetes playbook came up. As we talked more about it we both realized that even if you have the greatest book of plays ever assembled, and then you organize them neatly in a binder, the team that wins is the team that:

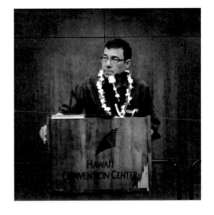

a) Did the better job of picking out which play to use in a given situation; and,

b) Executed the play.

Delivering the Sugar Surfing message at a recent TCOYD event in Hawaii. In addition to my own writing, Kevin's perspectives as a diabetes dad, diabetes technologist and behavioral researcher are reflected within.

Finally, the winning team must first be motivated and then prepared. In my experience this simply doesn't work in reverse. To be a winner takes more than just knowing numbers or knowing the playbook. Believing in your own self-worth and that you can do this is a great start.

Continuous Glucose Monitoring, or CGM, is a relatively new tool in diabetes management. Most doctors have received little to no training on CGM. Very few doctors know how to help patients with CGM let alone apply my new method of dynamic diabetes management. My advantage arises from my experience living with type 1 diabetes for almost 50 years, working with children (and adults) with diabetes for over 33 years, being a CDE (certified diabetes educator) for 25 years, and finally, using that insight and experience over the past 6 years while constantly wearing a CGM device. You will find few people on the planet who exceed these qualifications.

Through my recent journey, I discovered that there was a lack of good information available to explain the disconnect between my actions and my resulting blood sugar level. I learned that things I used to assume were hard facts no longer made much sense. As a result, I then began sharing my personal experience on the Internet. People's interest in my posts quite literally blew me away. So many kindred spirits coming together to share great questions, comments, and ideas led me to know that I wasn't the only one recognizing the disconnect between classic teachings and my new reality. Sugar Surfing was born!

I soon began giving talks and workshops about Sugar Surfing to patients, families, and health care professionals. As it turns out, online posts and comments are quite limited as a way to share knowledge. It becomes a hap hazard back and forth while jumping around from this and that. At many people's urging I agreed to write this book. It's still funny to realize that with all of the technology available for communicating online, the tried and true paper bound book is still hard to beat.

This book takes all of the best advice that I've shared in my free workshops, social media sites and my blog/website, and walks you through a carefully crafted instructional guide. My goal is to teach the reader how to apply the principles of Sugar Surfing to their day to day living; to give readers my strategy around when to apply one play over another. I hope to also surround Sugar Surfers with a supportive network of information as well as like-minded, knowledgeable people. I'm truly inspired by the support we received. The most important thing is how we feel about ourselves. It directly impacts how we navigate the daily minefields of diabetes care… and get up tomorrow ready to do it again.

Are you a Victim or a Victor? What shapes these feelings we hold inside? It begins with our personal biases. Much of what we believe to be true at diabetes diagnosis turns out to be myth and misconceptions.

If not careful we become lost in the fog or subject to the practice of 'Diabetes Voodoo' believing in things or techniques that simply aren't true. The sooner we release the demons of assumption the better. How we're treated or spoken to by loved ones, friends and acquaintances acts to either empower or enslave us. Guilt and fear erode self-esteem. The first step in Sugar Surfing is to toss those feelings overboard. Be prepared, embrace uncertainty, and kick diabetes butt!

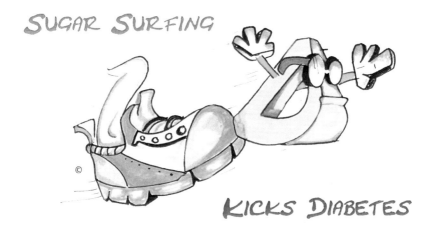

A Force for Change
Chapter 1

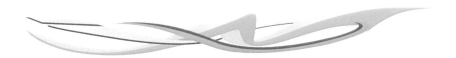

As a general rule, diabetes management has been taught as a set of "static" rules to follow. This way of thinking infers that a diabetes management action, whether it involves food, insulin, or activity should always yield the same result. Unfortunately, it's not that simple.

The insulin doses and meal plans assigned to newly diagnosed type 1 diabetes patients often come from published formulas, personal experience of the doctor, and published recommendations from diabetes organizations. On one level, these sources seem beyond question. But in the end they take little about you as an individual into consideration. Simply stated, they are just starting points. Because they work well for a time, they are rarely if ever questioned. This is one of the first origins of static diabetes management thinking.

Static diabetes self-care models are necessary at first. I dislike the fact that few type 1 diabetes patients ever get exposed to the true randomness of their condition and dynamic approaches to problem solving early in their education. In the era of CGM this stands to change. This book is my way of creating more discussion and making that change happen.

The human body is designed to adapt to change. Every major organ system we possess can adjust in response to changing conditions and circumstances. So why should our prescribed diabetes self-care be so rigid and resistant to frequent change? It is truly a fantasy that there is a one size fits all approach to diabetes.

Our response to insulin, food, and activity is not the same from day to day. It wasn't until I began using a CGM that I understood how many different forces there are which influence how our bodies respond. The boilerplate style insulin and food formulas I learned in medical school brought me close to realizing my full potential but still left me wanting more.

The ability to see the results of my diabetes self-care choices and actions in real time taught me a valuable lesson; that my bodily functions can be vastly different in terms of how they manage sugar levels day to day. Given that I've worked with thousands of people with type 1 diabetes and not just my own, I know that my experience is no different. There are only general estimates to gauge what our bodies need to best manage blood sugar levels. There is just no universal formula. What I learned was that I must discover my own unique blood sugar responses to food, activity, stress, and insulin and to be ready for all of these things to change all the time. The only way to really learn about my body's changing dynamics was to safely experiment, observe and create my own repertoire of responses.

With a CGM, I quickly learned that the classic "rule of 15", namely to treat a low BG with 15 grams of fast acting carbohydrates and wait 15 minutes to recheck the effect, often over treated my milder low blood sugars. Yet at other times it seemed to fall woefully short. Likewise, I found that my correction doses of insulin for a high BG would both

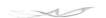

under and over-shoot their intended targets. Exercise also didn't always lower my BG and sometimes even raised it.

The only logical conclusion was that I had to discover my unique responses to food, activity, stress, and insulin, then repeatedly track them carefully with my BG meter and CGM device. While I could have done this with a blood sugar meter, the CGM made the journey of self-experimentation much easier.

Sugar Surfing then is a method which allows you to adjust your management style to best fit whatever situation you find yourself. Respecting the weaknesses of a CGM and knowing how to use it make my approach to managing type 1 diabetes practical and relatively safe.

Like surfing, having the right equipment and taking proper care of your tools is the foundation of successful Sugar Surfing. We will discuss how to get off to a safe and simple start. You will fall off your board. That is expected and frankly it's part of becoming a Sugar Surfer. Yes, wipeouts will happen as will the joy of a long smooth ride. More importantly, this book teaches how to fail safely while gaining invaluable experience. My hope is that what you learn here will make your future efforts more closely match your expectations.

Patience, Consistency and Resilience

I've found that well managed persons with diabetes (and most chronic diseases) possess what I call the "Three Virtues"; the first being patience. This virtue is especially valuable to Sugar Surfers. Since many of our medicines, foods, exercise, and stress have built in time delays, it requires us to be patient if we are ever going to learn what is truly happening inside. As it turns out, the actions you take and those that happen automatically operate on their own time schedule.

The second virtue of the Sugar Surfer is consistency. Develop a personal style or approach that can be reproduced consistently from situation to situation. Randomness is as pervasive in diabetes as it is in life. Consistency is refined through practice and lots of it.

This page has been sponsored by: Tyler Perez

The third virtue of the Sugar Surfer is resilience. This is the most sustaining trait. It speaks to one's own sense of determination and desire to succeed. It's an internal sense of strength that can often be seen by others and can be an ongoing source of strength for the one who possesses it. It's what often separates 'wannabes' from accomplished Sugar Surfers. It also develops from practicing the first two traits of patience and consistency.

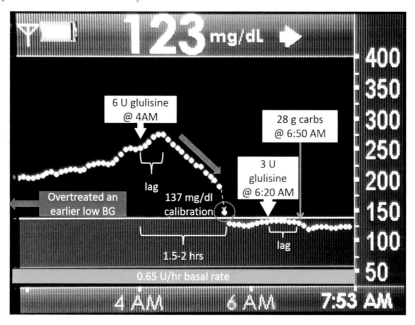

There will be liberal use of diagrams and illustrations like the one above to get you off to the best start. The comments I've made to images like this will show you how to interpret the BG tracings on your own CGM. Frequent glances at the screen on your sensor receiver, integrated insulin pump, smart watch, smartphone or someday soon even your TV or car dashboard will become second nature. But how well these data are used is limited by the skills and expertise of the user. That is the purpose of this book; to make you the best user YOU want to be.

It's important to understand that many forces drive blood sugar levels up and down within the bloodstream. The concept of Sugar Surfing is based on the acceptance of chaos in biological systems combined with the desire to make adjustments proactively and react to unexpected BG changes before things get out of hand.

"To improve is to change. To be perfect is to change often."

–   *Winston Churchill*

Our bodies must be able to quickly adjust to changing environments and life situations. Did you realize that your blood stream serves as both a delivery pathway as well as a waste disposal system? Under normal circumstances these two functions peacefully coexist and even complement one another.

In persons with diabetes, the major problem is the lack of ability to maintain "proper" or stable ranges of sugar in the bloodstream. For most persons with diabetes this is because of a lack of the hormone called insulin or lack of enough response to the insulin that already is present in the bloodstream.

Blood sugar or glucose is the primary energy source for large tissues and organs like the muscles, liver and the brain. In fact the brain cannot properly function without a sufficient level of glucose to fuel the high amount of chemical energy our brains demand from minute to minute. Anyone who has experienced low blood sugar knows how important glucose is for your ability to function normally.

Your blood sugar is constantly in motion. In most non-diabetic people there is a constant ebb and flow. Since these sugar levels remain within certain upper and lower limits we usually don't ever take much notice. But in persons with diabetes, sugar levels can shift and drift into higher (and lower) ranges more often, quickly and with seemingly little explanation. Unlike the tides of the ocean, blood sugar levels will drift and flux sometimes with little rhyme or reason. The truth is that in

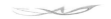

This page has been sponsored by: Trey Mize

many cases what happens to blood sugars can be predicted in advance and in some cases prevented or minimized. The key lesson here: "If it can be predicted, it can be manipulated".

One goal of diabetes self-management is to develop a working appreciation and understanding of these forces of change. Also, we aim to learn (over time) how to prevent or control these forces through personal decisions, choices and actions. You can reach your goal by making a conscious and determined effort based on constructive attitudes and principles. Not by engaging in reckless behaviors or making totally chaotic choices.

Until the person with diabetes is taken out of the decision making loop, which is still a long way off, the day to day blood sugar control of any person with diabetes is the sum of their actions and inactions. Diabetes control exists in the moment and is the product of what you do and those things you don't do.

For example, not taking medication or not eating are acts of omission that can have profound effects on blood sugar levels in persons with diabetes. It's important to focus on the things you choose NOT to do just as equally as you consider your measurable or observable acts.

In the grand scheme of diabetes self-management, I explain to patients and families that I (the doctor) don't "manage" anyone's diabetes. My role is more like that of a coach, occasional cheerleader, mentor, and at times role model I suppose. It truly is the sum of your choices; not mine or your doctor's. Simply receiving diabetes education is often not enough. I see a three step process at work, and often times we barely get past the first step. What we call "diabetes education" is intended to result in understanding on the part of the person(s) receiving it. But that is not the final element. Understanding should translate into behavior or actions for the education "loop" to be intact. There are many highly intelligent and understanding individuals in the criminal justice system who are well educated and understand all too

well their actions, even the illegal ones.

So what does all this have to do with using a CGM? In my opinion, it means all the difference in the world. It morphs a CGM device from a simple high or low blood alarm system (not a bad thing by itself) into the key for unlocking a vast new universe of diabetes self-realization that could once only be dreamed about.

Basic diabetes self-care can be drawn as a decision loop. This loop is actually being executed daily by most persons with diabetes albeit often in a mindless fashion. Turning this chore into a more mindful action loop transforms this into an incredible tool for attaining the best blood sugar control possible for you.

Like any loop, Sugar Surfing has no beginning or end. I tend to jump in at the point I call "monitoring". This embodies many inputs both measurable and subjective. Most of us think of the act of measuring a blood sugar level with a meter or CGM device. But it's more than that. It's also being "in the moment". That means being aware of recent, current and impending actions that are known to affect the ebb and flow of blood sugar levels in the body.

Since blood sugar levels can be unpredictable, staying "in the moment" is a about the only approach that works for anticipating, or at least quickly reacting to unexpected shifts in BG.

Once the status of the system (your body) has been sized up, either through the act of measuring a glucose level or glancing at the screen of your CGM device (or both), the next step is to analyze what is going on. This involves pulling in memories of recent actions (last insulin dose, most recent bout of exercise, what and how much was eaten (or will be soon) and more. The analysis step is where all of the little inputs come together for a final determination which is the next step: decision-making.

Deciding is prioritizing one or more actions based on all the possible actions. The one that seems to be the best option is placed at the top of

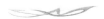

This page has been sponsored by: The Nightscout Foundation

the list to be acted upon. Back up options are most likely numerous, but an initial action is required.

The final part of our loop is execution: the act of following through on our decision. Immediately afterwards we are moving back into monitoring to determine the effect of our action and then modifying it as needed.

You are probably saying "I already do this" and you would be right. But as has been written about by many authors, many of our decisions are mindless as opposed to mindful. This loop is a skill as much as it is a process. And as such, skills are practicable and can improve over time, or grow rusty with disuse. For example, if you use an insulin pump, when was the last time you validated all of your built-in static ratios? This is what I call the cardinal sin of set it and forget it. If you find yourself simply acting on what your bolus wizard says then you are acting in a mindless state. Rather, be mindful and consider the pump's suggested bolus as simply another input to your decision.

CGM use is ideally suited for this four step cycle. Because the element of time and trends are inherently a part of how CGM data are visualized, it opens a new world of "glycemic calculus" which heretofore was limited to a static algebraic equation with little opportunity to shape or alter diabetes self-care actions until previous actions have already largely run their course.

I use the following metaphors to try and explain diabetes. I first remind folks that diabetes is a condition where the body can no longer maintain proper control of blood sugar levels. How one "gets" to that destination can be quite variable, even with the "type" that doctors like to assign a diabetes case. But diabetes "type" is just the tip of the iceberg when it comes to actual causation.

I can teach you the secrets of Sugar Surfing but you're the only one who can master these techniques. Now jump in, grab your board and let me take you to the beach!

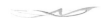

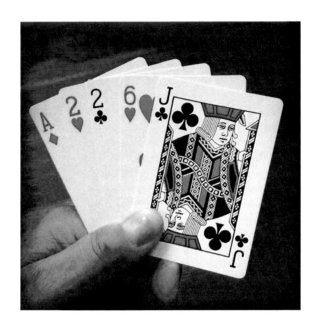

Bottom line, in diabetes, as in life, "It's not about holding the best cards. Rather, it's about playing a poor hand well".

- R. L. Stevenson

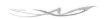

Why Am I Here?

Chapter 2

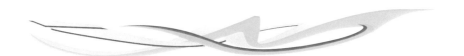

Recent medical studies have reported a 21 percent increase in the incidence of type 1 diabetes among children up to age 19. Over my thirty year diabetes medical career I can attest to this recent increase in membership to our exclusive club called type 1 diabetes. If you are reading this book, chances are you or a loved one, maybe your child or grandchild, is in the club. The increase in T1D prevalence was one reason I started my online education and support efforts; to reach more people touched by diabetes. We can meet this disease united or divided. You know where I stand on it. Each person is different and situations are different. This individualization is the basis of Sugar Surfing and why so many of you are Surfing already whether you call it that or something else. So now that you're here let me spend just a moment to help you understand some basics.

Diabetes is a condition where the body can no longer maintain proper control of blood sugar levels due to insufficient insulin. Insulin is a hormone required by the body to regulate blood sugar levels and make the sugar available to the body for growth and energy. With T1D, insulin by injection, whether via syringes or a pump, is required to manage diabetes.

With apologies to the game "Clue", the beta cells were killed in the pancreas by the immune system using cell-killing t-cells (not a pipe wrench or a candelabra). It's the "motive" we all wonder about. As we know, the poor hard working insulin producing beta cells don't want to bother anyone and quietly do their job every day. So why does our internal police force (the immune system) crack down on these guys so mercilessly? It's usually a case of mistaken identity, since parts of beta cells "resemble" a bad guy that the immune system is supposed to remove. Learning just how the immune police got this bad intelligence in the first place...and when... is the true research question that will someday allow us to exonerate the beta cells and get them off the immune system hit list and avoid their ultimate destruction.

Another metaphor I often use is "How many different ways can we get to Austin, Texas?" There are dozens of routes into this town and all will help you to arrive there. You may not know the precise route you took to diabetes, and you may never know the combination of biochemical events and missteps that it required. Of course we all like to speculate and I did too, but at some point I turned my mental energies totally to mastering my diabetes. I might not "like" my destination but I'm certainly obliged to learn my way around the city. You might call me a "city guide" who might show you how to navigate the best routes in 'diabetes town'. I certainly don't know how to build a road to exit this city. But I can help steer you away from the more dangerous parts of town.

Diabetes is diagnosed by abnormal blood sugar levels. These may also be called blood glucose levels, or BG levels. It's important to appreciate what "normal" means. In addition to classic signs and symptoms (increased thirst and urination), diabetes is diagnosed based on the following American Diabetes Association (ADA) criteria:

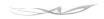

- A plasma blood sugar (after an 8 hour fast) ≥ 126 mg/dL (7.0 mmol/L);

- A 2-hour blood sugar level after drinking 75 grams of glucose in water ≥ 200 mg/dL (11.1 mmol/L); or,

- If someone with signs and symptoms has a random sugar level of ≥ 200 mg/dL (11.1 mmol/L).

   Note that non-diabetic persons can have RANDOM blood sugars up to 199 and be considered normal. Food for thought.

Definitions have become more strict over the years on the lower end. A fasting blood sugar of 110 mg/dL (6.1 mmol/L) used to be the upper threshold of normal until it was dropped to 100 mg/dL (5.6 mmol/L)over a decade ago. Under the right conditions any BG can exceed 200 mg/dL (11.1 mmol/L) in a non-diabetic person. It's why signs and symptoms are part of the criteria.

Blood sugar control is more complex than meets the eye and will change by a number of conditions or situations.

For example, my co-author, not having diabetes himself, investigated one of the early CGM devices prior to putting it on his daughter with T1D. At the time, he was a self-professed desk jockey and had ignored his own health in pursuit of developing a new tool to make school day management easier. What he found was surprising to him to say the least. With his new toy installed, of course he went to the "Golden Arches" and ordered up a giant burger, fries and a super-sized cola. And away he went. 120 (6.7 mmol/L)... 130... 140... 150... 160... He peaked at 167 mg/dL (9.3 mmol/L). All numbers were verified by finger-stick with a meter. While this was surprising to him, it's not atypical for people who don't have T1D to spike closer to 180 mg/dL (10.0 mmol/L) after a very large meal.

What is surprising is that his blood sugar only dropped into the 120s (6.7 to 7.2 mmol/L) and stayed there for approximately five hours before settling back into familiar territory in the 80s and 90s (4.4 – 5.5

mmol/L). And you wonder why you have a hard time keeping blood sugar from post meal spikes over 200 (11.1 mmol/L)? A few days later he confirmed a middle of the night low of 52 (2.9 mmol/L). Even the non-diabetic can have wild and unexplained swings in blood sugar.

"Normal" blood sugar levels in the absence of food or illness have a "floor" in non-diabetic persons: 72 mg/dL (4 mmol/L). This has been well-studied but of course like everything in diabetes there are exceptions. The body's first reaction as sugar levels drop below this level is a cessation of insulin release from the pancreas. Makes sense, right? As you can guess, this does not happen in a person with T1D.

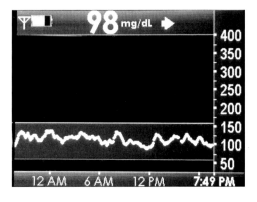

The chart above is of my non-diabetic daughter Rachel who also wore a CGM. As you can see, non-diabetics also have blood sugars that flux and drift.

The goal of diabetes management is to do your best to maintain an in-range blood glucose level more often than not, to minimize out-of-range blood glucose levels, and to move those inevitable out-of-range BGs back to where you want them.

Tired of dealing with "lows" yet? Low blood sugar in persons with T1D is believed to happen anywhere from 5,000 to 15,000 times in a lifetime. In most cases these lows are mild and properly self-treated. Only on rare occasion does the severe low BG happen. Unfortunately, these rare events are burned into our daily conscience and take up a disproportionate share of our memory.

While there is much we can do to keep our blood sugar from remaining elevated for long durations, we will experience high and low

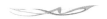

blood sugar. Of the two, low blood sugar is the situation requiring immediate attention and, to be honest, can sometimes take over my conscious and make me feel terrible. So, I do my best to minimize those kinds of lows, but no matter how much I try they still sneak up on me from time to time. Over my years with diabetes as well helping thousands of others, I believe that one of the biggest obstacles to living a normal life is "Fear of Hypoglycemia". It's a real problem for many parents and patients. Healthy respect for lows is totally appropriate, but fear has no place in being an empowered person with diabetes. Using insulin and having low blood sugar occasionally is not unlike giving knives to kids and expecting them not to occasionally get cut. It's a calculated risk, and we deal with that risk ahead of time by proper training on how to use a knife safely, coupled with the knowledge of what to do if it happens (preparation). So while we may remain vigilant and observe for proper safety, we don't spend each moment in fear. I have a good appreciation for what type 1 diabetes can and can't do to people. I've had my own brushes with severe hypoglycemia, too. Personally I choose empowerment over fear as the driver of my actions... and I try to promote that power within others. Try not to let fear and misunderstanding drive your agenda.

The body has lots of defense mechanisms against low BG. We all are at risk of falling prey to a post-traumatic stress syndrome-like situation after a severe low: patient or parent. This is magnified by the parent role and expectations we create for ourselves. I just aim to shine that light into an otherwise dark room to show that it's not always as scary as we make it out to be.

The body also has built-in protections against low blood sugar. Hunger is a biological defense against low blood sugar. However, food is not the only thing that raises blood sugar. As sugar falls further, the hormones glucagon, adrenaline, cortisol and growth hormone are sequentially released in an attempt to raise sugar levels through their different metabolic actions. In diabetes, we often artificially re-define what low blood sugar means. That doesn't mean the body understands. As a blood sugar manager, we need to get comfortable with adjusting

our definitions to meet the situation.

Likewise, correction of high blood sugars is important in diabetes management. While a low blood sugar may requires immediate action, unchecked or prolonged hyperglycemia has negative consequences as well. Knowing how to manage both is essential. This book will help you do just that.

As we leave this chapter behind, perhaps you will find a reminder of my basic 'Sick Day Rules' helpful. These tips should become second nature to you. They will aid in keeping any illness, infection, or pump malfunction from derailing your T1D control.

1. Check BG more often, not less;

2. Always check for ketones whenever sugar levels are over 300 mg/dL (16.7 mmol/L);

3. Treat high sugars aggressively with extra rapid acting insulin as needed;

4. Recheck BG (by meter) and ketones often;

5. Never omit a scheduled insulin dose. Illness usually demands more, not less, insulin;

6. Stay well hydrated with small sips of water or low carb liquids taken frequently;

7. Manage nausea early before it can turn into vomiting;

8. Become familiar with low-dose glucagon for raising those stubborn lows; and,

9. Call for help early rather than later.

Do what you can to help others and yourself, while you can. Appreciate EVERY DAY regardless of your personal health. And finally... Carpe diem!

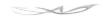

A Half Century of Diabetes

Chapter 3

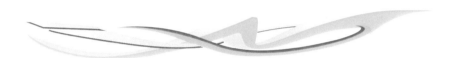

I was diagnosed with type 1 diabetes on March 1, 1966 after fairly mild symptoms: drinking a lot, 'peeing' a lot, losing a modest amount of weight… all the classic stuff. I was not in diabetic ketoacidosis yet I nevertheless stayed in an old-fashioned general hospital ward reserved for children (4 beds in a row) for 10 long days. Why ten days? The longer stay was thought necessary in those days to both "stabilize" my diabetes control and provide enough time to teach me and my parents how to manage my new condition. But I couldn't comprehend many of the concepts and medical words in the book and pamphlets we were given by my pediatrician.

My parents focused mostly on the daily tasks to be done more so than why or how things worked. Looking back as a 21st century physician, in 1966 there were few limits on how long a patient could stay in hospital. We had health insurance and most everything was covered and paid for without question. 'Care' was prescribed and the patient had little to no say over how things were to be done.

After I went home, my daily routine consisted of a single dose of insulin (called Lente) injected every morning by my Dad or Mom, plus several urine tests each day to look for sugar and ketones. A few drops of urine and water, then a fizzy tablet in a test tube which would make the liquid boil and churn. The color of the final solution was compared to a chart and then written down in a log book that my Mom made. The ketone test required a single drop of urine onto a small white tablet. If ketones were present in the urine the tablet would slowly change color from chalky white to various shades of purple based on the amount of ketones present. The ketone result was scored with a color chart by applying values ranging from negative, trace, small, moderate and large.

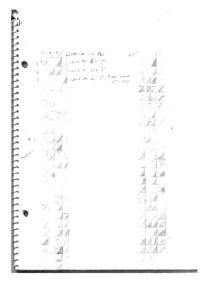

One thing I was not bothered by compared to today was numbers. All the measures of my diabetes control at home were based on colors and qualitative terms. I was spared seeing numbers throughout my childhood. Looking back, that might have been a blessing in many ways.

My diet consisted of a tear sheet the pediatrician gave my parents which had specific do's and don'ts. Total calories were 2200 each day, listed as food exchanges. Over the following years, the sheet was changed to 2500 and eventually 3000 calories a day. We never met with a dietitian during my entire childhood.

Disposable plastic syringes were more of a luxury then. Everything was reusable. Every morning my dad or mom would boil a glass

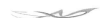

syringe (barrel and plunger) along with a reusable ¾ inch 25 gauge needle in a saucepan and strainer on the stove for about 20 minutes, then lay the items on a clean towel to dry and cool down before putting it all together and withdrawing my single dose of Lente insulin. Barbaric by today's standards, the glass plunger was prone to lock up, which meant the whole apparatus had to be removed and jiggled a bit (ouch). The needle would be used several weeks, being boiled each day of course. After repeated use the needles dulled (we were never taught to sharpen them). Such was life with diabetes 50 years ago.

My insulin dose was always the same, non-adjustable. My diet was supposed to be the same each day too but as I said my family never met with a dietitian during my entire childhood diabetes experience. All we had was that trusty tear sheet that got replaced with a slightly larger daily calorie amount as I got older and larger. At doctor visits the insulin might be changed a bit, but it was always just a single dose taken in the morning. That was my daily routine until 1981.

The late 1970's and 1980's ushered in the era of multi-dose insulin therapy and primitive insulin pumps. Having more "points of control" with insulin doses taken at meal time coupled with the use of a once per day long acting insulin to provide control overnight was believed to provide better day to day blood sugar levels versus once per day dosing of an intermediate lasting insulin (Lente in my case, like NPH).

It was around this time that the hemoglobin A1C test was developed. This test required a blood sample drawn from my arm and was analyzed in the lab. It gave doctors a way to gauge my past several months of overall diabetes control based on an estimated average blood sugar level. The results were provided as a percentage. Everyone has a certain amount of their hemoglobin bound to sugar, it's only a matter of how much. Non-diabetic persons have a low percentage of their hemoglobin molecules irreversibly bound to sugar (glucose). Usually, these levels range between 4-6% in most healthy people. As physicians, we rely on this test as a way to gain insight on how the patient is doing with their care and how well our prescribed medicines are working (or

not). However, this is only one of many factors physicians consider.

My first A1C test was done in 1980 and my result was 10.8. Other than the fact that it was higher than a non-diabetic value, it really meant nothing else to me. Not until later did I realize this value signified poor diabetes control. In 1983, I started using one the earliest insulin pumps; the Autosyringe MP-6. It was roughly nine inches long and was considered state of the art at that time. I bent the infusion needle at an angle so it would lie flat against the skin to be taped down. No infusion sets or plastic catheters were available then. Thankfully, the tools of diabetes management have improved by leaps and bounds, as has our understanding of diabetes management itself.

Moving Forward

By the 1980's, diabetes technologies were sufficiently developed to answer the scientific question whether or not "tight" or near-normal blood sugar control could slow down the development or progression of long term diabetes complications affecting the eyes, nerves and kidneys. This was finally put to the test in the landmark Diabetes Control and Complications Trial (DCCT) which reported its first findings in 1993. This major study showed that improving blood sugar control and keeping it controlled over time (about a decade) resulted in lower risks for long term diabetes complications or experiencing worsening of pre-existing complications. One of the measures that scientists tracked and controlled during this study was the A1C test. The goal was to lower A1C by 2% and sustain that level of control for 10 years.

The study was ultimately successful and proved what most scientists already largely suspected to be true: that closer to normal blood sugar levels are less damaging to the body over time. The study continues to this day under another name and follows the long term outcomes of all the original participants.

In the DCCT, the patients were between 13-39 years of age at the start of the study. They were psychologically screened for their ability

to be able to finish a ten year study, provided free supplies and medical care, plus were called by a nurse as often as once a week for the entire duration of the study. The 'intensive management' group was supposed to check blood sugar at least four times per day whereas the 'conventional' group would check zero to two times per day. These things had to be in place for study participants to be tightly controlled for 10 years. The average A1C for adults at the start was 9%. It was lowered to 7% during the study and maintained there. In teens, their starting A1C was about 10% and was lowered to an average of 8% during the entire study. Thanks to the results from DCCT, an A1C of 8% came to be considered one measurable definition of tight control for a teen over age 13. This study also showed that ANY sustained reduction in A1C was good for the person with diabetes in regards to lowering their RISK of complications or their progression.

There was also a dynamic element to the study. The DCCT medical team made changes in diabetes care as needed every week based on a standard set of questions and from manually recorded blood sugar logs provided by the patient or family. This couldn't have been more different than how my family and I were being taught to care for myself. After my diagnosis, little changed from week to week or month to month. My very first A1C in 1980 was 10.8%; about average for the time considering I took one injection a day and checked only urine sugars infrequently. In some ways my results were typical for the times.

Then in the 1980's and 90's came the rise of insulin dosing algorithms. These were based on formulas created by doctors observing well controlled diabetes patients and attempting to create a general formula for determining insulin needs. These formulas depended on careful observations by the patient of food to be eaten (mainly carbohydrates) and measured blood sugar values collected with the primitive glucose meters of the time.

This was definitely a step in the right direction toward individualizing diabetes self-care. But, these dosing formulas (which we still largely use today) often failed to provide consistent results.

What sometimes happened was that results indicating poor control often got blamed on the patient and not on the method itself since it usually worked most of the time.

The DCCT also helped to validate the use of insulin pumps and multi-dose insulin therapy as reasonable and relatively safe and effective methods to manage diabetes. Over the years, pump technology continued to improve and became easier to use: longer battery life, more reliable and precision electronics, convenient infusion sets, and faster insulin preparations. Insurance companies began (slowly) to provide coverage for pump therapy as well. We also experienced greater acceptance by patients, doctors and insurers for these intensive management techniques. Beginning in the early 2000's, these advancements contributed to the establishment of modern insulin pump therapy as we now know it.

In the mid-1960's the concept of measuring glucose (sugar) in living human tissue was conceived. It would be several more decades until the first practical continuous glucose monitors (CGM) would be available for widespread use. Today, CGM is an effective tool for persons with diabetes to use in making daily self-care choices. Several CGM companies have risen up while some have faltered. Many more CGM companies and tools are in the wings. Much like the adoption of insulin pumps a decade earlier, CGM is poised for rapid growth and widespread acceptance.

With the advent of blood sugar data provided in near real time, a new world of dynamic diabetes control becomes more feasible. Building on the success of CGM and insulin pumps, there is also a body of research attempting to create an 'Artificial Pancreas' (AP). The AP is a system that combines one or two hormone therapies to drive sugar levels up or down (insulin alone or insulin and glucagon in combination), a mechanized pump to infuse the hormones through a catheter(s) under the skin, and a CGM device to collect near real-time glucose data fed into a sophisticated computerized control system with the goal of completely managing blood sugar levels. The ultimate goal

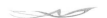

of AP researchers is to remove the user from having to make frequent self-care decisions but that is proving to be a lofty goal, indeed. At this writing, the future looks bright yet much work still needs to be done. The greatest downside may turn out to be the cost of maintaining such a system and whether or not insurers will cover the high ongoing expenses. Given the growing number of persons with insulin requiring diabetes worldwide, it's hard to imagine at this time that the AP will be a viable alternative for anyone except the affluent or those actively involved in the treatment side of research studies.

Meanwhile, currently available CGM already provides the opportunity for individuals to take a more direct role in their day to day self-care and in ways that they were never 'allowed' or taught to do.

Unfortunately, the development of new self-care methods and training to realize the full potential of these tools has been largely ignored, at least until now. For example, most CGM users are being trained to use CGM blood sugar data as a method to prompt the user to measure blood sugar by doing additional finger-sticks. While it's true that an old fashioned meter requires several minutes (not the test itself, but time spent gathering, performing and cleaning up). Compare that to a brief glance at your CGM readout which takes mere seconds. With more information in less time, tighter self-management becomes possible. And more improvements are underway to further streamline how quickly these data can be seen by the user, distant loved ones, the medical care team, or even devices equipped with forms of artificial intelligence. The future of diabetes management tools is wide open!

The Sugar Surfer's Manifesto

Chapter 4

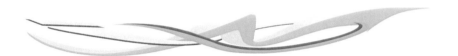

Sugar Surfing allows a person to understand how to make the best use of CGM or any other method of frequently collected blood glucose data. A CGM device reveals the cresting waves and shifting tides of human blood sugar levels throughout the day. This new approach provides a platform upon which to make thoughtful decisions about food, insulin, exercise and even stress management 'in the moment'. In fact, almost any of the ever present forces that influence one's blood sugar level can be managed with Sugar Surfing principles.

Sugar Surfing serves as a metaphor for dynamic diabetes management in contrast to what most of us have been taught; static diabetes management.

Surfing is something that can only be done well by a human being. A machine cannot be trained to Sugar Surf… at least not yet. The reason is straightforward: diabetes self-care is part reactive and part proactive.

Sugar Surfing embraces both concepts and weaves them into a dynamic model of care.

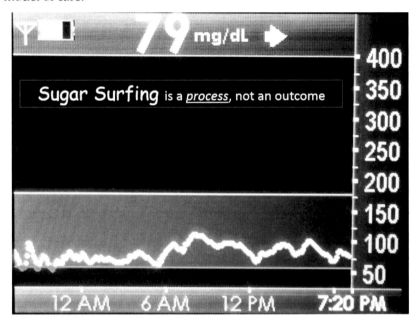

A machine can't predict human behavior from moment to moment nor can it reliably predict the future. The best any machine can do is respond or react. Our current artificial pancreas (AP) technologies still lag far behind a healthy working pancreas. Over time this will improve as AP's incorporate ultra-rapid acting insulin preparations to better match insulin to food as well as the possibilities available from a stable glucagon reservoir to reverse a trending low BG. Glucose sensors are still limited by a small lag time between what is measured in blood and under the skin (where current generation CGM sensors do their measuring) along with a host of other seemingly apparent barriers. Research continues into fully implanted glucose sensors placed deeper within the body. Some day, many or perhaps even all of these barriers will be overcome. However, until we are presented with a highly reliable and effective totally closed-loop AP, people will need to learn to Sugar Surf as a complement to blood sugar meters and CGM.

This page has been sponsored by: Ruby Morgan

To be fair, a pancreas can't really predict the future either. But it really doesn't need to. Due to its unique position within the body, the pancreas "sees" the nutrients we consume from food and drink as they first enter the bloodstream. Since it has insulin already produced and ready for immediate use, it can get jump ahead of rising blood sugar levels and release a proper amount of insulin to keep sugar levels from traveling too high after eating. It also possesses the ability to stop releasing insulin very quickly, almost immediately, to reduce the risk of low blood sugar. You might call it nimble!

Sugar Surfing blends the reactive and proactive abilities of human beings to manipulate the ebb and flow of blood sugar levels in response to a variety of different circumstances.

This brief history of diabetes management technologies and principles sets the stage for why this book has been written: as a tool to instruct and educate users of glucose sensing devices to empower themselves in the art of informed decision making.

Pivoting is at the heart of Sugar Surfing. I will discuss what pivoting is in greater detail later in the book. All your surfing skills are applied to make this happen. Much like ocean surfing, the longer you do it, the better you get.

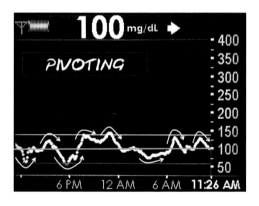

"Pivoting": In this case the middle of the range is 100 mg/dL (5.6 mmol/L). The high limit is 140 mg/dL (7.8 mmol/L) and the low limit is 60 mg/dL (3.3 mmol/L).

Where you set your personal target zone or zones is always you or your doctor's choice. When starting out, higher and wider ranges are always a good idea. As your skills

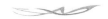

improve start to lower the target and maybe make the range narrower as you gain experience. A few words of caution: "Don't overdo it!" It's easy to make things too hard on yourself at first and often times you just can't keep blood sugars in range no matter what you do. We all have those days, including myself. They are nothing to be ashamed of. I consider my mistakes and missteps as chances to learn new things about my diabetes control. You should, too. When I checked into the mindset of tight control, I left behind any baggage of guilt and shame.

I respect my diabetes, but I no longer fear it like I did in my younger days.

There will be plenty of examples in the following chapters teaching you how to steer or bend your own blood sugars curves as you deal with flux, drift and other characteristics of dynamic diabetes management.

Over time, as my Sugar Surfing skills improved, I "zeroed in" my personal BG targets to a "pivot point" or "bull's-eye" of 100 mg/dL (5.5 mmol/L) with the low alarm alert set at 60 mg/dL (3.3 mmol/L) and high alert set at 140 mg/dL (7.8 mmol/L). My high-low alert ranges had originally started out wider and higher (pivoting at 150 mg/dL [8.3 mmol/L], alert range 70-200 mg/dL [3.9-11.1 mmol/L]). When you start surfing, aim higher and wider with your targets and ranges. Even so, I had to deal with some frequent high and low alert alarms at first. With experience I got better at setting the right targets and false or annoying alarms happened less often.

Whenever the situation calls for it, I adjust (manually re-set) my alarm thresholds to temporarily suit the circumstances. In the future, I imagine a more dynamic approach to alarms in these devices. I might widen them if I want to trend higher for exercise, or lower them if I want to be notified of a trending BG after a meal containing slow-acting carbohydrates. If you choose to temporarily readjust your personal BG alert thresholds, just remember to put them back to their usual settings. This will help to avoid annoying or missed notifications when things

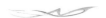

get back to your 'usual' routine.

Sugar Surfing calls for maintaining situational awareness. Changing your settings to match the situation will often result in early notification that can help you stay ahead of the curve as sugar levels trend up or down.

Sugar Surfing is a set of skills that anyone can learn. I can't overstate this. It takes patience, practice and perseverance to tame the "drift and flux" in blood sugar levels throughout the day. Sugar Surfing cannot be given to you as a formula on a piece of paper or settings programmed into your insulin pump. It's for these reasons that I always say that diabetes control exists "in the moment". My blood sugar levels are the result of things I do as well as things I don't do. In other words: my choices make the difference. Don't fall into the quicksand of static thinking, the infallibility of insulin and carb ratios determined months ago and complicated insulin dosing algorithms. Even the mobile applications now available for your phone are designed for static diabetes management. I discuss this in more detail later in the chapter "False Idols".

These tools may be good starting points. But, tightly controlling one's diabetes requires you to understand that nearly everything is almost always changing. Your blood sugar control is largely a matter of how much time you are able (and willing) to invest in it. Without your commitment to this process you may gain a lot of knowledge about Sugar Surfing but you'll have a difficult time "Going Pro". To be a successful Sugar Surfer you must be willing to:

"Look, Think, Act and Stay Mindful… Repeat!"

So you want to Sugar Surf? This book will take you through the following concepts and give you many practical examples and tips on how to perform these techniques to help you become a Master Sugar Surfer. What follows are the Six Keys to Sugar Surfing:

1. Know basic sugar surfing skills well; use them all the time.

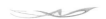

This includes keeping your CGM properly calibrated at all times, making sure your basal insulin (pump or by injection) is doing its job, learning the art of micro-dosing (insulin) and micro-carbing (fast acting sugar) and practicing the art of insulin-food "timing". I have a term for this one called "Waiting for the Bend": interpreting trend line inflection or bending points as they are happening in real time.

You will develop a level of comfort with between meal insulin dosing (with or without an insulin pump). You will learn that insulin dosing formulas or sliding scales are at best just starting points; nothing more. The same applies with counting carbohydrates in foods, too. There is just too much unpredictability baked into diabetes care. You must first accept it, then set out to manipulate it. Since most of us crave predictability and certainty, Sugar Surfing takes a little getting used to.

The act of balancing oneself upright on a moving surfboard, just ahead of a breaking wave, just above a sharp coral reef, riding for what may seem like an eternity… all the while being pushed by the incredibly powerful energy of a cresting wave… seems equally unnerving to the novice. You ride what the Sea gives you, not what you were expecting.

2. Develop the habit of frequent CGM display glances.

I suppose I look at my sensor readout more frequently than the average user, but certainly far less than a working pancreas (i.e. - continuously). I'm especially "visually vigilant" around mealtime, snacks, or after an insulin dose; times when sugars are more likely to suddenly and unexpectedly change. Viewing the BG data stream is one secret of your ultimate success as a surfer. Frequent feedback is your friend.

Knowledge of your blood sugar can translate into power over it. If you're not happy with the results (trending) you're

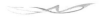

This page has been sponsored by: Raquel Manaois Gee

getting, try keeping track of how often you look at your CGM display. To be a surfer, you should expect to view your blood sugar status at least 20 times per day, and easily upwards of 40 or 50 depending on your day. Sugar Surfing is not necessarily easier. However, with frequent check-ins, you'll rarely have to dedicate three or four hours to correcting a glycemic crisis that's gotten too far out of hand.

3.   Set personal pivot points.

These can be flexible. You can move your own pivot points as you need to, based on the situation. For example, set a bull's eye of 150 mg/dL (8.3 mmol/L) to start. Set your upper and lower alarm limits wide at first. Just don't feel locked in. When starting out, aim for higher and wider targets. Your goal is to aim at steering most of your BG values well within your chosen range.

Pivot points are adjustable to the situation. For example, an athlete may desire higher target ranges during a competition. At different times of the day, ranges might be changed such as at night for younger children or for persons living alone. Nothing about this should feel revolutionary. After all, diabetes care is supposed to be individualized!

Hint: By making it easier to achieve targets at first with wide ranges and a higher pivot target, you will develop self-confidence. After all, your confidence is very, very important. Also, don't rush things. My journey to pivoting at 100 mg/dL (5.5 mmol/L) took a couple of years to achieve.

4.   Putting it all together.

As your CGM trend line moves away or towards your pivot point, decide which (if any) of your self-management tools are needed to change the direction. For example, as the trend line appears to move downward, select a point or situation when

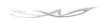

you will act in order to "bend" or neutralize a trending low blood sugar tracing. It's recommended to check your BG using your meter first before acting.

Experiment with different methods (a meal, snack, glucose tabs, juice, ice cream, engine braking, pump suspend) or a blend of different actions. You will learn about these later.

Similarly, if your BG is trending upward and away from your desired target or pivot point, decide if a sugar lowering force is needed, or just watchful waiting for things to turn around or level out.

Your options in these situations include insulin (as a standard pump bolus or injection), a "sleep bolus", combo or dual wave pump bolus, exercise, stress management, getting better hydrated, or some blend of all these things.

At first, just watching the trend line to get a feel for how your body operates under different circumstance may be your best first action. After all, a CGM device shows you things about your blood sugar that you never knew were happening: like sudden spikes from stress or excitement, drops from irregular insulin activity, or late-effects of exercise. Of course don't let things get too extreme in either direction before you act. A CGM allows you to first test drive your body's blood sugar system under normal routines. Relax. Observe. Learn.

Experienced surfers always study the waves before paddling out on the water to attack them.

5. Keep doing it!

And most of all don't expect perfection. As I say, "The only person with a straight line blood sugar is a dead person". Sugar Surfing is learning how to manage the slow drifts and rapid changes (flux) in blood sugar levels as reflected by the convenience of a CGM device.

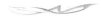

This page has been sponsored by: Piper Spradley

The magic of Sugar Surfing is developing the ability to steer and shape the direction of your trend line; in other words to make it work for YOU. But even when things seem to get away from you, your surfing skills are there to steer you back to calmer waters. If you're watching the trend line carefully, deciding frequently (whether you do anything or not) and then acting on your decisions, will translate into better blood sugar control in the long run no matter what the trend line shape looks like. And please remember to live each day one at a time. No surfer is perfect. The wipeout you had on Monday is behind you. Tomorrow you can be "hangin' ten". There are always new waves to conquer. Again, self-confidence is a huge key to your success.

6. As your surfing abilities grow, challenge yourself with lower targets, narrower ranges and situational pivot points.

That's the path to surfing excellence. Be careful not to overdo it. Diabetes is a marathon, not a sprint. My philosophy is to achieve a sense of physical well-being and "normalcy". Whatever you set as your personal goals, make them achievable and don't judge yourself harshly when you stumble or fall. Making mistakes just means you're human and that you're trying. The secret here is to learn from your mistakes whenever you can. You will see many of my own blood sugar mistakes in the following chapters. They paved my path to excellence.

Embrace your errors and become wiser from them. I'm confident you can do the same if you can be patient, consistent, and most of all don't give up. We are often our own worst critics. Give yourself a break. For me, the sense of control I feel over my diabetes is all the reward I need to keep doing this. The lower A1C levels (mid-5%) are just a bonus. I guess I'm a bit of a control freak but I do enjoy kicking my diabetes in the butt every chance I can get!

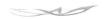

An insulin pump is not necessary to Sugar Surf

Some of us have a hard time being attached to anything for long periods of time: sensor or insulin pump. These feelings can keep some people from trying or staying with these devices. This is understandable. If you're getting technology fatigue, you might consider taking a CGM holiday every now and then, too. I took an insulin pump holiday for 3 years and wore just a sensor and used multi-dose insulin therapy. Most of us will put up with something if we believe it will be good for us in the long run. If you become impatient and expect surfing success to fall in your lap, you might not yet be ready to Sugar Surf. But if you've made a personal commitment to yourself and are willing to work through the obstacles life throws in front of you, be patient, persevere, and learn from your own mistakes, then you're ready to start Sugar Surfing.

Just the information streaming in to you from the display screen combined with your own experience and personal desire to stay in control is sufficient. If you take a CGM holiday, you might be quite surprised with the skills you've developed from using one, such as recognizing your own internal sensations of rising, dropping or in-range blood sugars as well as advanced trouble shooting skills having become second nature. Heck, even deciding to take a break from the sensor can be a useful experiment as long as

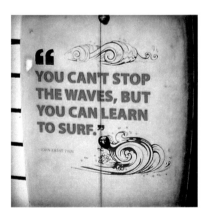

I saw this on a surfboard at Cocoa Beach in Florida while watching a surfing competition. I can't think of a better sentence that sums up the basic intent of Sugar Surfing.

you're willing to continue frequent blood sugar checks with your meter. Perhaps not 20 per day but as needed depending on the situation.

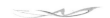

If you have diabetes and are internally motivated or driven, I feel Sugar Surfing is a natural fit for you. But even if you're not quite there yet, many of the basic principles I've discussed above can and will help you no matter where you're at with your diabetes care.

Despite what we're usually taught about type 1 diabetes, it's never really tamed. It's at best something to be managed "in the moment". There is no reservoir of "good control" stored somewhere, simply to be dipped into when things get difficult or challenging. Our diabetes control resembles a surfer riding the crests and troughs of a wave, navigating through its predictable and unpredictable elements towards a destination: the next wave.

Unfortunately, Sugar Surfers never get to 'call it a day' or head in when you're tired or you don't like the way the surf is breaking today. This is why you have to develop a mental toughness that is not only good for your diabetes but will serve you well in other parts of your life.

If you were to make your own list of things you control and compare it to the things you don't, it might look a bit like this:

Things I Have Direct Control Over

What I eat, when I eat, how much I eat, when I take my insulin, how much insulin I take, how I take my insulin and how often I take it, when I do activity, when I stop, how intense my activities are, when I check my blood sugar and when I don't, how I respond to the things that happen to me. This list could go on and on.

Things I Don't Have Direct Control Over

These might include: the actions of others, illnesses, Acts of God, the weather, and again the list could go on and on.

And there is an in-between list of things we don't have full control over but might still be able to influence somehow. Some examples might be how I react to the things that happen to me by others, how I

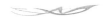

might attempt to change the actions of others and how I might best prepare myself for the unpredictable... or not.

I challenge you to make a list of the things you feel you control, the things you don't, and the things you have some ability to influence.

You might discover you have a lot more points of control than you realize, plus an ability to influence more things than you gave yourself credit. Why not take a few minutes to jot down your own control checklist. I guarantee that as you work toward becoming a Pro Surfer, your list will change.

Eclectic Diabetes Tools

I once composed a list of 'eclectic diabetes care tools' that I use. You might have many of your own that have been proven over time to serve you well.

You might find many of these quite beneficial. As you will read, many are situationally dependent. But regardless, these ARE TOOLS and should be recalled when the circumstances arise and they're needed.

Order of eating foods. If your blood sugar is trending high and it's about time to eat, not only will you aim to get the meal time insulin dose on board as soon as you can before sitting down to eat, but you can also consider changing the order of what you eat first. If you are eating a full meal, work on the salad or non-carbohydrate veggies or meal entré. This works in reverse too, but is more intuitive for most of us. When we are low, we will eat the fast-acting carbs first and take our insulin close to the meal. We must recall that meal time insulin takes at least 20 minutes to alter the uptake of sugar into cells, even though it gets absorbed by the body in 5-10 minutes. Insulin works best about an hour later (or longer). Timing is very important and can blunt a spike (up or down) in blood sugar levels. Arranging the order of the foods eaten can also be a helpful diabetes self-care tip.

This page has been sponsored by: Patrick Pappas

Stalling for time. This is a bit like the above tip, but takes things a bit further. If in a social setting and if your blood sugar is trending higher than you like, and you want to have time for the corrective and meal time insulin effect to start lowering your high reading, go socialize a bit longer. Find a topic of interest with your host that you can discuss freely and buy your insulin some time to show up for work.

Zig zag basal rate. This is a very unique use of a very low basal rate for small children on the lowest possible basal rate settings on a pump. It involves changing the basal rate every hour between the two lowest settings to get a value somewhere in-between. It can also be used to set a rate even lower than the lowest rate available. For example, if the rate is set for 30 minutes at zero, then on for 30 minutes at the lowest setting possible you cut that hours dose in half. This alternates all day 30 on, 30 off. It's a rarely needed tool, but works if carefully applied.

Chew your food. This is a vastly under appreciated tool. The process of digestion starts with chewing your food. Many of our processed foods are designed to be swallowed after only two to three bites. This means that there are large amounts of partially chewed food entering the stomach where they sit. And there it stays as stomach juices take their own time to break it down. Only then can the food get through the stomach and into the intestines where the sugar is taken up. This is one major reason there is a lot of irregular blood sugar levels even in persons who count carbs well. Chew your food if you want to eliminate one more variable and achieve a more predictable glycemic effect. It also helps in raising a low blood sugar that much quicker.

Drink water. This is based on a physiologic fact. The human body tries to rid itself of excess sugar by excreting it through the kidneys. We know that even in the total absence of insulin, if the body is well hydrated, the kidney can "pump out" sugar into urine up to a level of about 300 mg/dL (16.7 mmol/L). This assumes that kidney function is otherwise normal. This is the rationale behind drinking water whenever in hot or humid environments and blood sugar is found to be over 300 mg/dL. Just drinking water will dilute the blood sugar to a

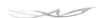

lower level, PLUS provide improved circulation to the tissues where an insulin dose is waiting to be picked up.

Dehydration reduces the effect of injected insulin by creating stress hormones that counteract insulin's effect, plus delaying proper absorption from injection sites, plus of course its diluting effect in the blood sugar level itself.

Drink your carbs. Most people think food needs to be solid to call it "food". Just remember that we all drink our food for the first few months of life, so this is a false belief. Liquid carbs can be in the form of milk or even some semi-solid foods like yogurt. When not in the mood for a solid meal, you can find suitable liquid alternatives these days. Don't discount their usefulness. They can provide a nice reproducible and measurable source of carbs compared to many solid sources, and often just as nutritious.

Fail safe. Keep carbs in the car (juice or tabs) and in purses and pockets. For years, I would make sure I kept money on hand to buy a snack if I got low. I didn't always remember to have fast acting glucose tabs with me. But as many would say, there are no carbs in a dollar bill. This tip is a great comfort-builder. Look at all the places you are, or the personal items you carry, and hide within them a source of fast acting carbs. Location examples include: 1) juice or tabs at the head of the bed or nightstand; 2) canned juice in the side pockets of the family car; 3) glucose tabs in school backpack pockets; 4) a juice source in the desk at work or school, as allowed; or, 5) a coat or jacket liner. Create a fail-safe set of surroundings and maintain them so that when you do have a developing low blood sugar event, it's short-lived.

Pre-dosing for highs before meals. If your blood sugar is high before a meal, and you know it in advance of the meal, it's perfectly proper to deliver a correction dose to get some insulin on board before eating. The correction and the meal time insulin don't necessarily need to be delivered at the same time. In fact, having a "leader" dose of corrective insulin could help ward off a spike later. Remember, the

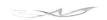

purpose of a corrective dose is just to bring you back to your target blood sugar level, plus or minus 30 mg/dL (1.7 or round up to 2 mmol/L) in most cases. Most kids on injections might not prefer this since it would involve two separate injections. Pumpers shouldn't care, but should remain vigilant to not forget to properly time and dose the remaining meal insulin later.

Keep supplies at hand when traveling. Insulin pens are easy to carry and store. You should carry your meter and a pen with you in an easy to get to location (coat, jacket, purse or backpack), especially when traveling. Protect them both from the extremes in temperature and discard as supplies start to age. Of course your fast acting carbs should be part of this kit. If traveling, make sure to carry on all your diabetes supplies or at least enough to get you to your final destination with extra to spare. Don't be a victim of missing or re-routed baggage!

Bolus tipping. This is an underused tool for insulin pumpers. It's how the pump bolus calculator can be used in reverse to determine the best range of carbs to consume to treat a low blood sugar. As you consume your obligatory 15 grams of fast-acting carbs, enter that amount of carbs, plus the blood sugar you just checked into the pump calculator. Don't give any insulin of course, but notice that it says NOT to take anything. Next, back out of the screen and reenter a larger carb amount and the blood sugar level. As you reach a level of carbs where the pump suggests some insulin to cover it, this "tipping" point represents the pumps best estimate of how many carbs to consume to effectively raise the blood sugar back to the target blood sugar on your pump. Of course this too takes practice and it also assumes that the duration of insulin action is activated on your pump and in a proper range. It's a great tool to prevent over treating a low when wearing a pump.

Super-bolusing. This is a pump tool that is very helpful for rapidly lowering high blood sugars or preventing blood sugar spikes with high glycemic index carbs. It involves stopping the basal rate for two to three hours and adding the equivalent amount of insulin to the bolus dose.

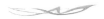

It's an advanced pump tool and highly effective if properly practiced and used sparingly. There is a good detailed explanation online by John Walsh. Google it.

There you go. These are just a few lesser used or "eclectic" diabetes self-care tools that more of us should consider using when the right situation arises. All require a good basic understanding of how they work, combined with a careful approach to their application. Practice also makes better. Just remember, we have many more diabetes self-care tools out there than we realize. Often, more than enough to get the job done well!

Remember...YOU are in control!

Sugar Surfing is based on a simple and profound principle: that YOU make all the choices that drive your diabetes one direction or the other. Your healthcare provider (doctor, diabetes educator, dietitian, mental health provider) can't make all your diabetes choices for you. They never have and never will. Advice, teaching and emotional support are all good things and very necessary, but in the everyday world diabetes "control" is the sum of our choices. This is a fundamental truth.

Sugar Surfing exists at the intersection of the educational, emotional and electronic elements of 21st century diabetes care. "In the moment" diabetes care has been searching for that final element. That final piece of the puzzle has now arrived: near-real time blood glucose "awareness" delivered in the form of continuous glucose monitoring. Without a CGM and in a pinch? Even meter checks every 20 minutes can give you the feedback you need to Sugar Surf during those intense short lived situations.

Remember that personal list of things you do control, don't control, and could possibly influence (under the right circumstances)? It's the tool kit of the Sugar Surfer. Make sure you take some time to create your list.

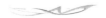

This page has been sponsored by. Nicholas & Jacque Privett

There are far more diabetes care tools at your disposal than you ever imagined. And by tools I don't mean meters, sensors, pumps, and the like. I mean the choices that you make, how you use these and other devices, the order in which you perform certain actions, and even knowing when and when not to act. Sugar Surfing is a skill to be learned and then practiced constantly. Your skills will grow and mature with time and experience, allowing you to develop newer skills you never imagined possible.

Thinking in a new way

Sugar Surfing asks you to often set aside your old, static ways of thinking. When first diagnosed, we are all introduced to formulas and pathways which direct our choices. Often there is no wiggle room whatsoever. In fact when we "ask" for some autonomy, or independence we are often met with a firm "No. Do as I say" with an implied "Or else". This sets us up for one of our first conflicts: going off the care plan given to us by our diabetes care team. Let's admit it. Say it with me now; "I cheat".

It could be eating more (or less) than we were told, not checking a blood sugar, checking "too often", not applying a ratio to calculate an insulin dose, ignoring what your pump "Wizard" has to say about dosing, having a piece of candy instead of a four gram glucose tab, a larger order of fries, omitting an insulin dose, or not exercising. There seems to be an infinite number of ways we can go off script. But whatever it might be, the end result for many of us is to feel guilty or to be accused of being a "bad diabetic".

Sadly, many of us don't simply fall into this trap, we are pushed into it. Our providers deliver a strict set of do's and don'ts along with perhaps a superficial, brief explanation as to why this is necessary. As patients, we expect our doctors to have our best interests at heart. After all, these people spend years getting trained, right? I will attest here that the majority of doctors I know DO have their patient's best interests at the core of their being.

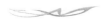

Static thinking dominates diabetes care

The problem for some people in the medical profession is that their training in the management of patients may have come from a "see one, do one, teach one" approach inherent in the health care. And depending on who they were trained by, might have adopted attitudes and behaviors about persons with diabetes that often carries a lot of negative assumptions.

The static method of diabetes control is easy to teach compared to dynamic diabetes management and most believe there is no other way to safely teach newly diagnosed persons. We need to embrace the dynamic method as soon as we can reasonably do so. That is one aim of this book.

So, new diabetes patients typically get their basic training not unlike how new military recruits go through boot camp. While everyone needs this entry level exposure, the experience hardly makes them ready to be Generals of their own diabetes destinies. This is where the health care system often fails persons with T1D. Since type 1's are in the minority (fewer than 10% of all persons with diabetes worldwide have T1D) many of the beliefs and attitudes these providers show to patients with type 2 diabetes are transferred to the person with type 1.

Finally, doctors can fall into a trap of generalizing too much in how they treat diabetes patients. New patients to my practice have told me of previous diabetes providers who had become inflexible and prescribed mostly boilerplate approaches to care. Given the large number of persons with diabetes in the world, it's not hard to imagine that many may feel burned out and have embraced a routine of dispensing "Care by Numbers". In such a black and white approach, you can see how promoting individualized care can be the first casualty.

We don't have enough fingers to point at the numerous reasons why there is room for improvement in how type 1 diabetes patients are taught and supported. And in spite of all of the progress I've witnessed

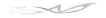

since I was diagnosed in 1966, there is a large and constantly growing group of persons who have received nothing more than a brief boot camp education, struggle to use anything but the most basic features included in their many diabetes devices, and find themselves lost and without good direction or support.

Many diabetes patients follow their provider's directions the best they know how, develop many myths and misconceptions about their own diabetes, and carry a lot of unnecessary guilt and fear about their condition. Sound familiar? If so, this book is written for you.

I don't want to end this chapter on a down note. There are many great diabetes professionals out there. These folks are dedicated and passionate people who routinely go "over and above" for their patients. I'm very fortunate to work with many such individuals now and many others in the past. These people empower, enlighten and inspire their patients…and me!

Well, there it is: *The Sugar Surfer's Manifesto*. These principles and skills will be discussed and described carefully in the following chapters. But surfing success? That's up to you. Like everything else in Sugar Surfing, it's your choice now whether or not you turn the page.

False Idols

Chapter 5

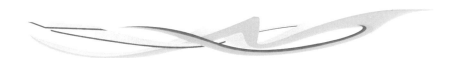

In order to move from purely static teachings about how to manage diabetes, a person needs to embrace the idea that much of what they have been taught has been grossly oversimplified. If you believe this statement is too strong, then just consider how much of the diabetes basics we're taught are riddled with exceptions, inconsistencies, and nuance. This chapter's theme is to point out that just about everything in diabetes self-care we've been taught as constants, are at best, only estimates. This idea will strike many as heresy. But as a doctor who also trains other doctors, I can attest that many providers in the healthcare field struggle with the ambiguous nature of working with persons with type 1 diabetes. Don't think static thinking is only a challenge for patients to grow beyond. The medical profession needs to move ahead in their thinking as well.

The good news is that our ability to handicap and estimate the forces that influence our sugar levels can be exercised much like a muscle. It just takes the right mindset. In the late 90's Sci-Fi thriller "The Matrix", Neo is confronted with a pivotal choice early in the plot of the film by his mentor Morpheus. When Neo is told that the world around him is nothing more than a computer generated fantasy and that he can choose the true reality and perhaps rewrite the course of history, Morpheus extends his open hands holding a red pill in his right palm and blue pill in his left.

"This is your last chance. After this, there is no turning back. You take the blue pill - the story ends, you wake up in your bed and believe whatever you want to believe. You take the red pill - you stay in Wonderland and I show you how deep the rabbit-hole goes."

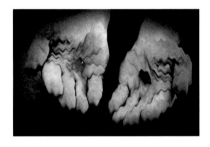

If you've read this far, it's now time for you to make a choice. If you wish to see the world of diabetes as largely black and white, utterly predictable and capable of being managed well by only a few simple actions each day, then put this book down and go back to whatever you were doing. But if you choose to explore the true diabetes Wonderland with all its inconsistencies and contradictions, then read on.

How many of us truly realize that the numbers which seem to be everywhere in the management of diabetes are merely rough approximations and not commandments inscribed on a stone tablet? What numbers? How about meter results, carbohydrate counts, insulin doses, insulin correction factors, insulin to carbohydrate ratios, and A1C results, just to name a few. Diabetes is overrun with numbers. And with numbers comes a tendency to judge; often too harshly. We become our own worst critics which mostly serves to hold us back rather than move us forward.

Because of our vulnerability and lack of knowledge, skill, and emotional stability when we're first diagnosed, we rarely question the

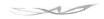

numbers that are assigned to us. And we're taught to embrace each of these numbers as if they exist in discrete and separate bubbles (e.g. X + Y always equals Z). How the numbers are determined may not be explained by your doctor, but given to you as a set of rules to follow.

Factors common in the first year or so after diagnosis (regaining lost weight and the end of the "honeymoon" phase) usually result in a gradual need for more injected insulin to maintain adequate blood sugar control. Then to make it worse, many practices instruct the patient to never give a correction dose of insulin unless blood sugars exceed 250 mg/dL (13.9 mmol/L) and only at the planned meal time. Such a conservative approach is felt to be in the patient's best interest at first. But like wet concrete, these instructions often harden around the patient or family's feet leaving little to no flexibility as time moves forward. This is how the static thinking invades our perspective and in so many ways.

Could there be a better way to handle this transition? Of course. But how could a remote medical team possibly teach one newly diagnosed patient how to do this on their own and safely, let alone hundreds. Herein lay the beginnings of the "false idols" (myths and untruths) that are so common in diabetes. If you've managed diabetes for any length of time at all you either get extremely frustrated and depressed while clinging to these static numbers or you begin to understand that there is a pervasive flaw with trying to control blood sugar using 'Diabetes by Numbers'. I prefer to call this Static diabetes management.

This chapter is critical for anyone considering a switch to Dynamic diabetes management or what I call Sugar Surfing. For those who find it hard to let go of Diabetes by Numbers you will struggle as a surfer. Anyone who has ever body surfed or used a boogie board knows that there are some things you must leave behind when you begin to learn how to surf. For example, if you hold on to the comfort of the prone position, close to the water with a low center of gravity and are hesitant to pop-up on your new surfboard, it will take you much longer before

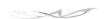

you get to experience the thrill of a long ride with a clear view of the beach.

Over the next several pages many of these myths and untruths will be exposed. Knowing that much of what we've been taught needs to be at least questioned, marginalized or dismissed entirely is critical for your success as a Sugar Surfer. For many, simply understanding that these numbers are merely guides or starting points and that you need to test their validity often may be the breakthrough you need. With this new perspective, the artificial barriers placed in front of you by false idols can be avoided. And make no mistake; these idols have been in place for decades created and perpetuated by well-meaning people in positions of knowledge and authority (myself included). They too have become comfortable with these idols and continue to light candles around them to help show you the way.

It's not that what we teach diabetes patients is necessarily wrong. Rather, it's incomplete. To explain all the exceptions as a rule or guideline is being explained, or a new technology is being taught to a user, can quickly become overwhelming to a person who is relatively new to diabetes. But given how poorly we educate persons with diabetes overall, at least beyond the basics, it's easy to see how we aim to help the most people by keeping diabetes teaching methods focused on simple actions and concepts. In essence we tend to oversimplify, often to an extreme.

Furthermore, many patients with diabetes may not want this flood of information and nuance at first. They might find it overwhelming, confusing, and overrun with medical jargon. Some patients may struggle with understanding basic health issues based on their personal, educational or cultural background. If you're not careful, embracing these false idols will keep you from realizing your aspirations of a more normal life. In no particular order, I present to you the "False Idols" of diabetes:

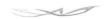

This page has been sponsored by: Mike Barry

Carb Counting

One basic principle of medical nutrition training (MNT) for diabetes is to attempt to quantify (or at least regulate) the average amount of carbohydrates, fats and protein consumed each day, based on each meal and snacks. Carbohydrates are largely converted (at least 90%) into sugar (glucose) by the process of digestion and absorption in the intestines. Smaller percentages of fat (3%) and protein (7-10%) can experience a similar fate. Carb counting is based on the premise that it's best to focus on tracking carbohydrates and allow greater latitude with fat and protein in certain situations. This should not be a license to disregard these two other macronutrients since they do contribute calories (4 calories per gram of protein and 9 calories per gram of fat) and can affect other aspects of health.

So, learning the difference between fats, proteins and carbohydrates is an important step in managing blood sugar. Fats and proteins tend to slow down the digestion process in part by controlling how quickly the stomach empties food into the intestinal tract. This is why foods with a combination of macronutrients (carbs, fat and protein) may affect the rate of change in blood sugar differently (slower) compared to whether these macronutrients are eaten by themselves (e.g., pure carbs). At first, some persons tend to think a meal is a meal is a meal, but that perception quickly changes when one starts to look at the differences in blood sugar responses that might follow even when meals are thought to contain identical amounts of carbs, fat, and protein. Fat and protein are broken down by the digestive process into their basic building blocks and used for growth, cellular repair and other vital bodily functions. Carbohydrates are used largely for energy (sugar) but also provide substances for numerous bodily functions. The reality is that we require all three macronutrients to survive. The relative percentages of each that we consume daily is a topic of active debate and I will not take part in that discussion in this book. Low-carb, low-fat, low-protein and everything in between have their vocal advocates in books and online. Sugar Surfing can be done in all these scenarios, but you must

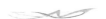

be aware of the glycemic effect of the foods you put into your body if you expect to be a quality Sugar Surfer.

Nearly everyone can utilize simple sugars (e.g. - juice) in short order whereas "complex" carbohydrate foods like pizza, some pastas, and most foods with high proportions of fat and protein combined with carbs, will generally digest much more slowly and deliver sugar to the bloodstream in a more gradual and extended fashion. It's well known that pizza can take several hours to complete the process of conversion to glucose. And it might be further complicated by what is being consumed with the pizza including the toppings (pineapple?), sugary beverages, a salad with fatty dressing and even how well the food was chewed.

The act of chewing is the first step in digestion within the body. Saliva contains enzymes which begin the digestion process, and chewing starts to break larger pieces of food into smaller ones. Once in the stomach, this process continues, aided by powerful stomach acids and enzymes. The process of cooking food is also part of the digestion process. Heat applied to foods starts to break down the chemical structure of food, making it easier to breakdown and digest. This is why equal amounts of a rare steak may deliver fewer calories than a well done steak, since a portion of the rare steak may never get broken down enough to be completely absorbed by the intestines.

The concept of carbohydrate counting could lead some to believe that eating can be a science. That might be possible in a clinical research lab, but in the real world, carb counts are estimated at best. Factors beyond the actual amount of food eaten will influence how the body breaks down and absorbs the food or meal.

A study done a few years ago with type 1 teens involved thoroughly teaching them carbohydrate counting skills using the foods they preferred to eat. Then after just one month, when these same teens were tested to demonstrate their proficiency, less than one quarter of them could accurately count carbs within 10 grams of an assigned food that

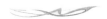

they preferred to eat. Few persons will ever get the extensive training those teens received as part of that study.

I'm not being dismissive of carb counting. On the contrary, I attempt to quantify the carbs in everything I eat. But I just don't stop there. I realize that even if I read a label or weigh a portion, my body's blood sugar response may respond to that food differently from day to day, or even from meal to meal. I'm also careful not to become anxious over this step and quickly come up with my estimate. I use carb counting as a starting point, not as the final answer. If I guessed incorrectly my surfing skills are there to help me catch the next wave.

Only through personal experimentation will you be able to avoid surprise lows and highs that can be associated with this inherent variability that is simply part of eating food and drink. My aim is to avoid or minimize mismatches between my insulin action and the entry of sugar into my body based on the rates of conversion of the mixture of carbohydrates, fats and proteins in the meals I eat.

Hopefully you have access to a diabetes education program with a skilled dietitian experienced in teaching how to best estimate (count) carbs. Hopefully you get to see this professional as often as you wish to learn this important skill. However, just like we were taught about the reliability and constancy of insulin ratios, we need to understand that carb counting is a necessary but hardly infallible skill due to all its "baked-in" variability. If you've found yourself perplexed with inconsistent blood sugar responses in spite of meticulous carb counting efforts, you've gotten caught up in applying the principle of precision thinking to things that are inherently imprecise. That is a recipe for frustration. Sugar Surfing can free you from this.

"How many grams of carbohydrate are in an apple?" How big is it? What kind? How ripe? How big is the core in relation to the total size (the part you don't eat)? Teaching someone how to accurately and precisely count the carbs in an apple would be a very difficult task and would take many hours of training. For someone who is highly

sensitive to insulin, just being off by 10% could result in a significant swing in that person's blood sugar.

Perhaps a better approach is to think of food in terms of Estimated Food Impact (EFI). Because there are so many variables in play around food, why not think of that food as part of a situation rather than only a specific number of grams of carbohydrate. Things to consider when coming up with an EFI for that food event include: a rough estimate of the grams that will convert to sugar; the speed at which this meal or snack will convert to sugar; how quickly is my blood sugar rising or falling based on CGM (which may need to be verified by finger stick); if blood sugar is high, how long has it been high; and many more considerations.

So, take your best shot at counting carbs, estimate your insulin needs including the situation, take a bolus from your pump or give yourself an injection, and here's the important part: study the impact of your actions using a properly calibrated CGM! I can't stress this enough: You are far better off to simply monitor and manipulate blood sugar movements rather than obsess over calculating the accurate number of grams of carbohydrate in a given apple. If in doubt about what or how much you will eat, you may always take a smaller "leader dose" of insulin to get the process of sugar disposal started. This will be discussed later.

I use the following metaphor to drive home the fallacy of insulin ratios and carb counting as stand-alone tools for tight control.

What would you say to the golf pro that told you "All that's required to find the green is a) choose the right club, b) grip it properly, c) maintain the correct shoulder stance, d) keep your eye on the ball, and e) shift your body weight properly as you swing through the ball. If you do these things you will always find the green and just maybe… a hole in one"?

Your first thought should (appropriately) be "You're nuts"! So why should we believe a spot blood sugar level plus a measured amount of

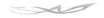

food (carb counted) plus an insulin dose from a static formula (e.g. your insulin pump 'wizard') will consistently result in an in-range blood sugar level 2-3 hours later? That's nuts!

Basal insulin

It's common to hear persons with type 1 diabetes say "I want to get back into better control" or "I need to get my insulin dose regulated". Both statements suggest that diabetes control is a place to go to or that there is an insulin prescription that is just right, and we just haven't found it yet.

Basal insulin is a great example of static thinking. Insulin pumps are programmed to give the same rate profiles each day unless the user changes something, such as applying a temporary basal rate. But even this is rarely done unless under a doctor's direction and even then, it's done infrequently (such as during illness). But the basal insulin needs of a person are constantly changing from day to day even in good health. This is well known and not new science.

Insulin pump therapy seems to encourage static thinking given its need for stored ratios. Think about it this way; the body does not have a quota of insulin to deliver each day, it simple responds to the needs as they present themselves. Even basal insulin needs drift up and down each day based on circumstances not under anyone's control. Illness, medications, stress, sleep disturbances and changes in activity levels will influence the amount of insulin produced between meals and snacks in non-diabetic people. This is yet another reason why blood sugar levels don't travel along a straight line in non-diabetic persons.

In the world of Sugar Surfing, the basal rate is like everything else: just a starting point. It's not the end all and be all many believe it to be. It too requires daily attention (in the form of CGM trend checks when glancing at the readout) and at times daily adjustments to keep the BG trend line within your target range.

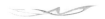

This page has been sponsored by: Megan G. Davis

If basal insulin delivery by injection or insulin pump consistently causes upward or downward drifts in BG in the absence of food, activity or stress, then changes to those doses or settings are usually needed. But failing to appreciate the imprecise nature of basal insulin often leads persons down a path of making frequent basal insulin changes which makes matters more complex without any significant improvement in overall BG control.

Insulin to Carbohydrate Ratios

How are you feeling today? Is your gut healthy or under stress? This affects the absorption of nutrients and thus to what degree the carbohydrates get broken down and absorbed into the bloodstream. The intestines are in essence a large sheet of biological tissue capable of absorbing the products of digestion. In other words, taking substances from outside our bodies and moving them inside our bodies. Any condition or disease that affects the stability or size of that large sheet can have a temporary or permanent impact on what gets into our system.

Some persons with type 1 diabetes also develop celiac disease. This condition is caused by an allergic/autoimmune response to the substance gluten found in many natural grains. If poorly treated, celiac disease can reduce the absorption of nutrition from the intestines by flattening the villi, those little fingers that line the small intestine, thereby exponentially increasing the size of that absorbing sheet. Undiagnosed or improperly managed celiac can result in inconsistent glycemic responses to food. But many other intestinal disorders can also affect how the gut absorbs things.

Short-lived conditions like viral gastroenteritis and other diarrheal illnesses can temporarily damage the gut's ability to absorb nutrients. This effect is fortunately temporary. There are many instances where the intestines can interfere with the predictability of food on blood sugar response.

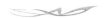

This page has been sponsored by: Maxi DeLedebur

There are also many variables in play when it comes to the relationship between insulin and food. Unfortunately, I feel the medical establishment has unwittingly done a disservice in attempting to simplify such a complicated facet of diabetes self-care. With too much emphasis on drugs and machines and less on education, coaching and long term support, we have taken a very expensive (and in my opinion misguided) path to the management of diabetes from a population standpoint.

In truth, insulin and carbohydrates are constantly moving targets. Even your body's ability to make use of the exact same foods has been proven to be different from day to day.

If you don't believe me why not try this little experiment. Take a loaf of bread, a tablespoon of peanut butter and a tablespoon of jelly. Weigh each of these so you can be sure that you have the exact same amount of the different nutrient profiles. Also, don't forget to calibrate your weight scale before you weigh your food.

Plan to eat your sandwich at the exact same time on both days and try to have your blood sugar within 30 points or so when taking the challenge. I think you'll find that you get different results. Go ahead and try the challenge again but this time eliminate even more of the variables from day to day. You can see that what I'm suggesting can easily be described as unhealthy behavior, and that is the point. We have all been taught that adhering to formulas is the key to better control, yet in order to make the formulas work we can easily become obsessed with the minutiae. And no matter how hard we try, the results will often times be different.

Why not give yourself a break and commit to learning how to surf? That freedom is called Sugar Surfing and it requires you to manage in the moment. It also requires you to rely on your memory a bit as snap decisions can be aided by recent memories of how you dealt with similar situations and what those results were.

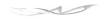

This page has been sponsored by: Max Hatfield & Joan Mead

Insulin Delivery Devices

This idol comes in a few different forms. One for those who use an insulin pump, another for those of you who give yourself multiple daily injections (MDI) by syringe and yet another for those who use an insulin pen.

For you pumpers, did you know that each pump is unique? Not only do pumps vary between manufacturers and model numbers, each pump is slightly different than the one that came off the production line before and after. Machines change and degrade over time, which may change its performance. Are your pump settings being regularly calibrated and inspected to ensure that the manufacturer's standards are still in effect? We do this for our vehicles every year. Yet, we have insulin pumps that take a beating every day and we only worry about replacing them when they completely break, or when 4 or 5 years have passed so insurance will pay for a new one. How crazy is that?

If you don't use a pump then you're on MDI using either an insulin pen or syringe. These are machines, too and have variance built in as well. Ever had a "wet shot" where some of the injected insulin sneaks out after you remove the needle? This can easily happen if you're not careful, and sometimes even when you are. Unfortunately, there are so many injections over the years that many fail to look for this potential confounder. They just inject and forget. User error comes into play on a regular basis, not because you didn't try, but sometimes that injection just didn't go as planned. Remember to look as you withdraw your syringe and if you see that some of your insulin is making a break for it don't stress. Just keep in mind that the near future is now ripe for higher blood sugars than expected. Because your Surf Wagon has many tools in it besides insulin, you can add in an activity or adjust your meal to match that lost insulin.

So when you wonder why corrections don't always result in bringing you back to your target, my advice is to move on and take another view toward your next step. Far too much time and energy is

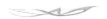

wasted on wondering vs. doing in the realm of diabetes self-care.

Duration of Insulin Action (DIA) – (aka: Insulin on Board (IOB) and Bolus on Board (BOB).

Regardless of how you get your insulin, insulin works differently from day to day even in the exact same setting. In some people, '24 hour insulin' only lasts 16 hours on one day but 22 on another and 26 hours on another. Some may experience a spike in the insulin action using a long acting insulin as opposed to the straight line effect most of us were taught.

Insulin delivered through your skin must traverse a gauntlet of obstacles to reach its final destination: your individual cells. Assuming the properly measured amount is taken, enzymes (insulinases) located in the skin start to degrade insulin as soon as it's injected. Also remember that a lot of kids (and some adults) forget their meal or snack doses altogether, take them late, or deliver an incorrect dose. Once insulin reaches a small blood capillary and gets whisked into the bloodstream, it's taken directly to the liver, which destroys a large and variable percentage of what gets delivered. After passing through the lungs and back to the heart, the insulin gets pumped out to the body where it eventually comes into contact with individual cells. These cells possess special receptors on their surfaces which bind to the insulin and set in motion a series of chemical reactions which result in specialized molecules called glucose transporters to move to the surface of the cells. It's through these transporters that sugar (glucose) is able to move into the cell and be used for energy to power all cellular functions.

As you can tell from the tortuous path that insulin takes, there are many locations along its journey where it can be destroyed. It's estimated that about 90% of a subcutaneously (through the skin) injected insulin dose is inactivated by the body before ever reaching its target destination. Some days are better than others and more or less insulin reaches its final destination unscathed. But the point here is: variability rules.

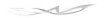

Other variables affecting insulin uptake involve the temperature of the skin at the injection site, the location of the site (arm, abdomen, leg, hip), the rate of blood flowing through the site itself (like an exercising body part), plus tiny differences in the depth of the injection. Other factors like smoking or dehydration will influence (slow down) how insulin is absorbed from an injection.

The amount of insulin injected will also tend to influence how long it hangs around. Larger doses of rapid acting insulin last longer than smaller doses. The same can be said about longer acting insulins.

Modern insulin pumps allow the user to automatically estimate how long an insulin dose is expected to be able to keep lowering blood sugar after that dose is delivered. This programmable value is called the duration of insulin action. If the pump "remembers" how much remaining insulin action is present since the last bolus dose, it can remove or subtract insulin from a later dose if that dose falls within the period of time when another dose may be needed to correct an out of range blood sugar level or "cover" an extra amount of carbs eaten. But since the DIA is a number, we're immediately at risk for becoming trapped in static thinking mode. The DIA is just an estimate, and it is often assigned based on assumptions made based on age or even the brand of insulin being used. Sugar Surfing allows for ways to determine the duration of insulin action using a CGM device and careful observations of the trend line after the insulin dose is given.

When deciding upon the duration of insulin action time to program into a standard insulin pump, the doctor may apply a middle of the road estimate such as 3, 4 or 5 hours. These values can and should be confirmed by careful BG trend line checking with a CGM. A future chapter will show you how using Sugar Surfing can help you to "see" what your DIA is on any given day. This forms the basis of the I-chain maneuver using insulin injections to emulate a combination or extended bolus function when eating a meal with complex or slow digesting carbohydrates.

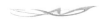

Numbers

Too many numbers, indeed. Driving is a funny thing. Every once in a while I look at the speedometer but I can pretty much tell how fast I'm going by watching the other cars around me or how quickly trees pass by. My car doesn't have a 3D directional indicator like you would find on the dash of an airplane. I can make tiny adjustments on the fly. If I'm drifting right I gently nudge the wheel to the left. If a ball rolls onto the road in front of me I hit the brakes or steer around it. I'm a successful driver because I'm paying attention to all of those little (and big) things around me all the time. That's why I don't need numbers to drive.

Similarly, there are no numbers in surfing other than the score a judge gives you. Yet surfers are able to manipulate the immense power of the ocean to create awe inspiring drops, bends, turns, aerials and yes… wipeouts. With the aid of a CGM and situationally appropriate guide rails, I can easily see how I'm doing in relation to that imaginary line that runs down the middle of my wave. Most of what I'm doing becomes second nature.

But alas, numbers do become necessary in diabetes. Insulin doses are numerical and blood sugar levels are as well. I sometimes wish we could go back to a color based approach from my childhood. Red zone, green zone, blue zone, yellow zone, etc. Aim to stay out of the red zone and more in the green. Colors between green and red could emphasize need for lesser actions to steer the sugar levels back into green. Sound far-fetched? Perhaps, but it might be associated with less angst and guilt based on the judgment that comes with numbers.

Numbers remain a necessary element of our care but they should not overshadow the intuitive aspects of our self-management.

Calibration

Machines that determine values typically require a process to compare the result from the machine to an outside reference standard.

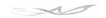

The process of adjusting that machine to match the reference standard is called calibration. Many modern timepieces are calibrated to the atomic clock. In diabetes, calibration is supposed to be performed by the patient. Rarely is this done. Blood sugar meters come with control solutions to test the accuracy and quality of test strips. Less than 7% of meter users ever use control solution. But even if they did, there is tremendous variance in the accuracy of commercial blood sugar meters, even under ideal circumstances.

In the USA, the Food & Drug Administration has a process for allowing blood sugar meters and test strips to be sold to the public. The current FDA guidelines allow variance in the reading on the meter from what a highly accurate laboratory analyzer would report on the same sample. If the actual BG value is over 75 mg/dL (4.2 mmol/L), acceptable values from the meter could be 20 mg/dL (1.1 mmol/L) above or below the actual value and the meter would still be considered acceptable for use by the public. If the BG was under 75 mg/dL, the variance must be 15 mg/dL (0.8 mmol/L) or less (that's a 30 point range! [1.7 mmol/L]). Finally, in 5% of test cases, the value can deviate from the actual reading by ANY amount. There is a movement afoot to tighten up these variances but for now realize that this false idol is real and account for the possibility that the number you see is only a ballpark estimate.

And none of this takes into account poor BG testing technique on the part of the patient (e.g. unwashed hands, barely large enough sample size, squeezing the finger and alternative site testing among others). I'm not even counting those times when your child gets a friend or the family dog to offer up a sample of their non-diabetic blood to cover up that piece of cake you said "No" to. These data are being used to make decisions about self-care by the patient and at times the doctor. Plus, these same data are used to calibrate a CGM device. The reality is that commercial blood sugar meters provide estimates of blood sugar levels. Just try repeating BG checks several times in a row and see how variable the results can be.

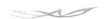

This page has been sponsored by: Marlen Gutierrez

This doesn't mean that modern BG testing is worthless. The results obtained from a properly collected sample are still very useful for individual use and sufficiently accurate for calibrating current generation CGM devices. The take home message here is that care must be practiced in the collection of these data. And, if the meter result is inconsistent with the situation, always question the meter result before questioning the situation. In other words, don't hesitate to repeat a blood sugar check by meter when your senses tell you something is amiss. Make sure you read Chapter 6; "Waxing Your Board".

Hemoglobin A1C

Like blood sugar meters, did you know that even the best office based A1C analyzer machines have leeway or variance in their accuracy and precision? For example, when you are given a number, that result can be +/- 10% of the true result. Further, studies show that with the point of care A1C analyzers, the ones that give results in minutes using just a finger stick blood sample, your result can be more than a half point off when compared to the result obtained using the same sample on one of the most accurate laboratory analyzers.

Unbeknownst to you, your A1C blood sample may be analyzed in a different lab, using a different method, on a different lab analyzer and by a different lab technician. All of these differences may contribute to meaningfully different results.

On a positive note, there is now a method that helps standardize A1C results from different methods based on an internationally accepted standard. This is now being adopted in most major laboratories worldwide. However, the point of care A1C analyzers are not included in this change.

The moral of the story? Don't get too hung up on whether or not your A1C went up or down by a 0.3. That kind of difference is easily within the acceptable variance of the technology and may have very little to do with how hard you worked at managing blood sugar. Yet, we smile or cry when we see or hear that the A1C went down or up by

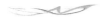

even as little as a half point. A better use of that number is to assess what you did to influence the A1C and how your actions contributed to those results within a wider range of the spectrum. For example, an A1C of 7 vs. 9. As a surfer, your experiences in the moment far outweigh the importance of a single number on your quarterly report card.

Maybe we should bring the use of colors into the discussion here, too. Each 1% change in A1C could be associated with a different color scheme. Unfortunately, I witness too much unnecessary anxiety over minor differences in A1C which can be easily explained away by the sheer variability inherent in the laboratory analysis process. For example, a child's A1C which apparently goes up from a 7.8 to 8.1 is somehow interpreted by some as 'being a bad parent'. Where this guilt comes from I do not know but color reporting might eliminate a lot of this anxiety and senseless guilt. More food for thought I suppose.

Basal Profiles

How many different profiles do you have programmed in your insulin pump? When was the last time you tested your basal profile or dose? What is going on with the ratio between basal vs. bolus as a reflection of your total daily dose? In other words, do you really think that your body is the same day in day out or might there be some wiggle room here and there? Absolutely! For starters, if you have six basal profiles, why not try to see how you do with only five. The reason is that the more variables you remove from the equation, the easier it is to predict what might happen in the future. Studies have shown that fewer basal rates leads to clinically significant improvements in outcomes. Simpler is better!

The reason for so many basal rates can be traced back to how many doctors think. When I was a static thinker, I would look at BG patterns and make changes to basal rates rather than spend time addressing insulin dose timing or what was being eaten. Since doctors are authorized to prescribe, that's what I did. Looking back, I was seduced

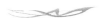

by the idea that changing pump settings was the answer to most problems. Plus patients might have thought something constructive was being done. I do think I helped in many cases, but I was not really addressing all the things that contributed to the BG patterns I saw.

Today, I advise patients that a basal rate (whether by pump or by injection) is intended to maintain stability in BG trends… mostly. If your 8 basal rates allow you to maintain a steady BG track in the absence of food, day after day, then that's what you need. But I rarely find that to be the case. Fluctuating basal rate delivery via a pump can be a major contributor to overall variability in blood sugar profiles.

Personally, I've evolved to using a single basal rate in my insulin pump. Now that might not work for everyone, but I advise anyone using a pump to keep the total number of basal rates to the lowest number necessary to maintain stability whenever food is delayed or omitted.

Glycemic Index (GI)

This is yet another number to consider when deciding the impact of a given food on blood sugar levels. Low, medium and high glycemic index foods convert to sugar at variable rates of speed. It's more helpful as a qualitative tool than a quantitative one. This is an extension of the fallacy that goes with relying too much on accurately counting carbohydrates. For example, when someone quotes you a GI for an apple, the best way to interpret this is how quickly it might raise the sugar level. The actual glycemic index value assigned to the apple would not help you much with calculating an insulin dose for it. Especially if you are combining that apple as a topping on your ice cream, sautéed in butter and smothered in cinnamon and nutmeg. A better approach might be to look at meal and snack time with an eye toward all of those things that need to be considered before taking a preemptive or corrective action, which may or may not include a dose of insulin.

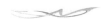

Insulin Dosing & Delivery

No matter how you get insulin inside your body, the tools we use are not entirely accurate or precise. There is always acceptable variance in the manufacture of plastic vessels, tubing and syringes. Insulin pumps have an acceptable variance when told to bolus a specific number of units. Did you know that when you use your insulin pump to bolus 1 unit of insulin it can be off by a range of plus or minus 30% - 200%? In relation to the powerful effect of a small dose of insulin, even small variances from shot to shot or pump bolus (including basal delivery) can have a meaningful impact on resulting blood sugar.

As to battery operated machinery, do you ever notice a difference in the performance of your electronics as the battery level goes from full to empty? Why would medical devices be immune to the Law of Variability?

Tunneling is a phenomenon of leakage of insulin around the edges of an infusion catheter outward towards the surface. This creates loss of expected insulin, is often unnoticed, and contributes to unexplained insulin responses. I've used Sugar Surfing to suspect and successfully identify tunneling in the past.

Air bubbles in tubed insulin pumps is another source of blood sugar variability that often goes undetected. This is best addressed by careful reservoir loading and proper priming of the infusion set before catheter insertion. Also, an occasional visual inspection of the tubing for bubbles or large air gaps can avert a case of hyperglycemia or worse.

Insulin action

Some people assume that injected insulin has the same action every time it is injected. This is false. There are multiple factors that impact insulin action. This applies to all types of injected insulin. This variability is discussed Chapter 12; "Surf Safely" and throughout the book.

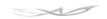

Fractional Unit Doses

In the mid 1990's at a medical conference, I met Dr. Paul Davidson from Atlanta, Georgia. Paul has been a pioneer in the field of clinical use of insulin pump therapy. In the 1980's he and his colleagues asked some very important questions regarding how to properly calculate insulin doses using the pumps of that era. Back then pumps were not enabled with calculators as they are today.

Dr. Davidson and colleagues had developed mathematical models to estimate insulin requirements for meals, corrections and basal rate determinations. In a short time, his ideas had earned widespread acceptance. But I had noticed that more and more patients were taking his concepts further than they were originally envisioned. For example, using insulin to carbohydrate ratios parsed to the decimal point.

Personally, I found this obsession with ultra-precision in insulin dosing a bit unnerving since I didn't usually see any improved control in patients who practiced it. When I mentioned this to Paul, I was struck by his response. He said that his basic dosing formula algorithms were never meant to be anything more than basic starting points for proper dose selection.

The way they had been morphed into decimal-point calculations was bemusing. I saw this as a good idea taken to an extreme. Certainly not by its creator, but by an eager and willing diabetes pump wearing patient population ultimately searching for a sense of certainty in a world of chaos.

This phenomenon is alive and well today and has become part of established diabetes practice. Much clinical research has been dedicated to parsing these insulin dosing formulas to their most sophisticated forms. Insulin pump manufacturers have even expanded their dosing accuracy to two decimal places if nothing else to differentiate their newest pump. Yet when these formulas are applied to the free-range patient (outside the clinical lab), they still constitute a static approach to care.

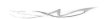

This page has been sponsored by: Jocelyn Hruby-Dodd

Day to Day Variability

It's true that there are high and low tides within the body for many hormone systems. These can influence blood sugar levels and response to insulin. Growth hormone, cortisol, estrogen, progesterone and testosterone can exert direct or indirect effects on blood sugar levels. But like much of what you've read about so far, these hormone surges are not as predictable as high and low tides in the ocean. Plus their impact does not occur in a vacuum. The variance in insulin, food, stress, illness (if present) and exercise all muddy the waters of predictability. But there are situations where hormonal high and low tides can be incorporated into Sugar Surfing strategies. So, understanding and appreciating their existence is very important.

One old Greek saying goes "You can never step into the same river twice because new waters are always flowing over you". This best summarizes how an experienced Sugar Surfer approaches the waves of sugar washing over her. In the Surfing world, each new wave is and will always be, unique.

Insulin Pumps

Insulin pumps have been around in some form since the 1970's. I've worn a pump for over 3 decades. I've also seen a mythology arise around pump therapy that almost rises to the level of a minor religion. Social media fans the flames of pump mania, too. Sometimes persons with diabetes get treated by other persons with diabetes as second class citizens because they don't have an insulin pump.

Don't misunderstand me, insulin pumps can be a positive force for better diabetes self-management, but they can be equally destructive and disempowering if improperly prescribed. Years ago I coined the "12 Commandments of Insulin Pumping", the first and most important of which is "An insulin pump is no better or worse than the human being attached to it" (or operating it). Pumps are no panacea. And a pump is not necessary to Sugar Surf. I used basal-bolus (injected) insulin therapy for 3 years as I developed the Sugar Surfing method to

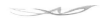

make this point.

Insulin pumps are also prime targets for misuse. We were all teenagers once. So I know that if there is a way to beat the system or "stick it to the man" I'm gonna do it just because I can. Well, an insulin pump is not foolproof. I won't get into the many ways to beat the system here as I liken that to sending a pickpocket to prison. They went in knowing how to take a wallet and didn't know how to not get caught. A year in the clink and they come out with a degree in crime. Bottom line, open communication and a team approach can't be beat for people managing type 1 diabetes. If you have a child with type 1 diabetes, frequent unannounced review of the pump history, oversight of insulin injections, frequent review of blood sugar history and discussion around meal time decisions are some of the best tools for helping your kid with diabetes. Don't think that buying them a $7,000 USD (nearly 5,000 GBP) machine and all the appurtenances is the answer all by itself. Type 1 diabetes management takes work.

Wizards

Now consider the bolus 'Wizard' commonly found in insulin pumps or in your favorite mobile app. Those calculators use ratios that were setup once upon a time by you or your diabetes educator or perhaps even a company representative. How much follow up has there been to confirm that these ratios are accurate or even to see how good you are at estimating carb counts? I think they should have expiration dates attached to them like everything else.

Can we all agree that the so-called insulin pump wizards are no more Wizards than the man pulling levers behind the curtain? Even though Dorothy in "The Wizard of Oz" should have known better, it took Toto to draw the curtain and expose the truth. I think we would all be better off if we stopped referring to machines and computer programs with magical qualities but rather call them 'calculators' that are also programmed to draw elements of a mathematical equation from a static repository of user (and physician) initiated variables'? Ok,

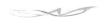

so wizard is sexy and a lot easier to say but I fear that sometimes people become so enamored with technology that they hand over the decision making, too.

Several people who have really taken off with Sugar Surfing have shared that one result is that they are far less interested in what their pump calculator has to say. It might still be a helpful input to your otherwise complex decision making process but your mind works much quicker and with more inputs than entering estimates of numbers into a static calculator.

Alcohol wipes don't eliminate sugar

Alcohol is not a cleaner. It is a disinfectant. One very important rule for proper use of a blood glucose meter is to wash your hands with soap and water and to make sure your finger is dry before lancing to draw a blood sample. When you use an alcohol wipe you are merely moving dirt and sugar around on your finger until the alcohol dries. If there was sugar on the finger before there is certainly sugar on the finger after. Also, if the alcohol is not completely evaporated it will denature the blood sample and skew your result. Try your best to wash your hands with soap and water before you check blood sugar using a meter. You can then skip the alcohol swab step altogether.

Quarterly Visits with Your Physician

Insurance companies typically won't pay for more than four hemoglobin A1C tests per year for those diagnosed with type 1 diabetes. Coincidence? I think not. For years the only way a physician could know how a patient was doing was to order an A1C test. There are standards for A1C results that also help providers to easily categorize their patients as 'well controlled' vs. 'poorly controlled'. So, when do you need to see your diabetes team? I suppose you need to see them when you need to see them and of course that depends on the quality of your care team and what issues you might be having at the time.

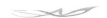

My advice to you is to commit to managing every day and in the moment. Don't cram three months of daily care into a few days of preparation for your quarterly visit. If you need motivation and a method for simplifying daily care then be glad you got your hands on this book. Read on future Sugar Surfer!

Peer Advice

It's not fair to compare. Taking advice from peers with diabetes or even people without diabetes is a recipe for frustration. First, the non-diabetic peers will advise you of all the cures and latest treatments they saw on TV or read about in the Good Housekeeping or Time magazine. They might ask you why you can't take a pill or ask you if it's alright for you to eat that food when dining with them. Second, diabetic peers might tell you how they can do this or that and still maintain great blood sugar levels.

Here's a classic example: cinnamon. Have you heard of that one before? Have you had a well-meaning friend tell you how some new supplement evens out the blood sugar spikes? These pitches come and go and never seem to be accompanied by solid research to support their claims. Peer advice can be helpful but it can also be harmful. Be sure to consider the source of the advice before putting it into action.

It's well known that type 1 diabetes patients can still produce insulin for years after diagnosis. Honeymoon phases can also extend for longer than a year for many persons. Some long term patients produce small amounts of insulin for decades (called micro-secretors). The exact meaning of this remains unclear, but what is clear is that no two persons with type 1 diabetes are completely identical. It's why I advise against general statements for all patients. Individual results may vary, as a famous tagline goes.

High Blood Sugar

There are just about as many largely arbitrary strategies for dealing with out of range blood sugar values as there are doctors to prescribe

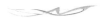

This page has been sponsored by: Maggie Rauschenberger

them. Some may choose not to treat as discussed earlier, others may be much more aggressive. The methods for determining how much insulin to give have been based on formulas. Hopefully they were further refined and improved by actual observations of their effects. But in the end they are still static in nature. As a provider I aim to avoid high blood sugar but as a realist I know that they will happen. I make every effort to provide tools for patients to correct an out of range single point blood sugar value or CGM trend.

Diabetes management is much more an art than a science, and with major psychological overtones. As much as the medical profession and health insurers might want it to be a predictable science, it won't be that for a long time, if ever.

"Never stack insulin"

This is addressed in Chapter 12 - Surf Safely.

"Never correct out of range blood sugars between meals"

In a recent meeting of diabetes educators, we were surprised to once again hear of entire programs recommending no action for blood sugar up to 250 mg/dL (13.9mmol/L). Patients are supposed to wait until their scheduled meal, check blood sugar and use a "sliding scale" issued to them for adding insulin to their scheduled insulin with a dictated carbohydrate meal plan.

In a static world, I might be able to partially defend this practice. Avoiding a between meal correction eliminates the need to teach critical thinking skills, especially if there is little BG testing being done by the patient. But this argument falls apart in the dynamic world of Sugar Surfing where BG trends rule.

Ordering people to ignore their instincts to correct high blood sugar is simply wrong. It has the potential to create all kinds of strange behavior, stress and complications when simply teaching patients how to safely correct out of range blood sugar using insulin has been broadly taught and accepted. If your care plan includes no corrections

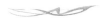

for high blood sugar you would be advised to question your provider or at least ask them to clarify their rationale so that you can fully understand it.

Biologically, this makes little sense too. In 1987 it was shown that the human body produces on average 11-12 waves of insulin from the pancreas each day. This is actually consistent across all persons without diabetes. I'm not advocating 11-12 insulin doses a day, but if non-diabetics produce insulin between meals, then maybe learning how to do that properly isn't a bad idea.

"Never Correct at Bedtime"

For many, a good night's sleep can last 8 or 9 hours. For kids and teens even longer. So why is it ok to let blood sugars run free-range for 40% - 50% of the day? It seems to me that if you're going to work so hard for the 12 hours that you're awake, you ought to have a game plan for dealing with the other 12 hours, too. Your target BG levels can and should be higher during sleep, but there are safe ways to correct a high BG at bedtime or midnight with less risk for a middle of the night low. There is a method called the Sleep Bolus for correcting high BG levels overnight. It's discussed in Chapter 12; "Surf Safely".

Perfection

Perfection is a concept created by humans, not a biological nirvana to achieve. Get rid of this mindset. There is no room for perfection in Sugar Surfing. Just look at a 24 hour CGM tracing of a non-diabetic person and you will see no straight lines. This relates back to the toxic nature of numbers used in diabetes management. If all you hear from your doc (or loved ones) is that a high BG is "bad" and an in range value is "good", you've been set up for a life of recurrent failure since even the best managed persons with diabetes will have an out of range reading at some time or another. The concept of perfect in diabetes care is a mirage. Find satisfaction in a job well done rather than attaining a specific numerical BG target. After all, the number you get may itself not be the exact true value, but most likely it's close enough and living

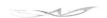

in a desirable range is far more satisfying than attaining a specific BG value and keeping it there. Even pro surfers in search of The Perfect Wave will tell you that the moment you finish that ride, you realize that there is yet a better wave in your future. If it's anywhere, it's found in the moment. You can't bank perfection.

3 Shots per Day

Stuck on the idea that you are only going to inject X number of times per day and no more? As I said above, the pancreas of a non-diabetic is known to unleash 11 internal insulin bolus events per day. How can you expect to have the blood sugar profile of a non-diabetic if you're not even open to the possibility of giving yourself half that many injections? Too busy to bother bolusing for that snack via your pump since it's a pain? "I'll just wait for dinner and correct then". But now you've set yourself up for the diabetes roller coaster. Major swings, major corrections, over corrections, reactions... when all you really needed to do was take a few minutes to properly deal with the situation up front.

What have you been taught about diabetes as if it were a sacred truth? How many of these 'false idols' have you already discovered? Are they affecting your current diabetes care? Have you managed to replace these idols with something that actually works? Hopefully, the chapters that follow will give you a more effective toolset than myth and misinformation.

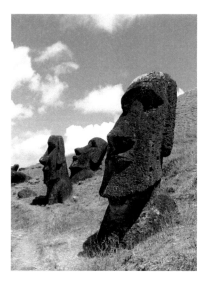

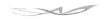

Waxing Your Board

Chapter 6

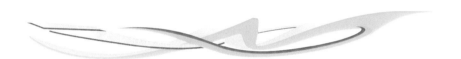

Calibration is key to successful Sugar Surfing.

Sugar Surfing in its purest form requires anywhere from 20 to 50 blood glucose inputs (assessments followed by a subset of actions) per day to fuel the decision making process. I consider each BG reading I collect from a BG meter or a glance of my sensor readout as a "pearl" of tremendous value. However, the relative value of this pearl of information is fleeting or ephemeral. I must choose whether or not to act on that information quickly or else its value is forever lost. This is why I believe diabetes self-control exists "in the moment".

You can't surf very long wearing a blindfold. BG checks and proper CGM calibration are an everyday requirement for successful Sugar Surfing. Essentially, you could Sugar Surf with only a meter but it's highly unlikely unless you're pathologically obsessive compulsive given the high number of meter checks you would need to perform each day. In short bursts, you can practice Sugar Surfing with a meter alone but I wouldn't advise trying to become a full time surfer with just a meter. Therefore, we'll assume for the rest of this book that you're using a CGM. In order to Sugar Surf, you must have a good "surfboard" and it needs to be prepared each time you head out. That means excellent ongoing calibration. This chapter teaches you how to do just that and why it's so important.

A common reason I hear from some persons who wore a CGM and then later stopped is "It's not accurate".

Modern CGM devices don't directly measure blood sugar levels. They do measure sugar (glucose), but it's the glucose that's located in the liquid located under the skin; also known as interstitial fluid. Glucose in the fluids of our body exists in different concentrations depending on the location. For example, the sugar level in the blood is higher than the levels in the liquid that bathes our brain (cerebrospinal fluid), inside the eye (called aqueous humor), or within a joint (called synovial fluid). But in each case, the levels are proportional to what is present in the blood. It's this basic principle which makes current CGM technology feasible as a tool to manage diabetes.

A CGM measures blood sugar levels indirectly. Inside the sensor tip is a tiny probe where a chemical reaction occurs. The reaction generates a small electrical current that is proportional to the amount of glucose in the fluid that comes into contact with the probe tip. The transmitter attached to the sensor receives the electrical signal and sends the information as a wireless message to the receiver unit (either separately held or as part of an insulin pump) every few minutes.

The process of calibrating your CGM is not unlike calibrating a bathroom weight scale. You take an object of known weight that is in close proximity to your own weight; say, a 150 pound bag of rice. Place the bag on the scale and then use a knob to adjust the scale until the scale matches the known 150 pound weight of the bag of rice. This is known as calibration.

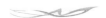

In order to make sense of what the CGM probe's electrical signal means, the system requires a periodic blood sugar reference (from a standard blood sugar meter device) to compare to. In other words, when the CGM signal reads "x", the BG at that moment is "y". The process by which the CGM is taught to match up these signals is also called calibration.

Proper sensor calibration is a core principle of Sugar Surfing. Reliable information from the sensor is crucial to making the best "in the moment" decisions and choices. And while current CGM devices continue to improve in regards to accuracy and precision, much of a sensor's reliability depends on the commitment and skills of its user. Training about this aspect of sensor use is often grossly under appreciated. It's related to the idea of "garbage in, garbage out".

Many CGM users don't appreciate how important it is to properly calibrate their devices. I personally know many diabetes patients, some doctors with diabetes and some diabetes educators with diabetes who wear CGM devices and calibrate their units in a haphazard fashion.

Common examples of shoddy CGM calibration include entering a false (made up) BG number into the unit when prompted. Some users report simply re-entering the BG value displayed on the sensor unit at the time the device requests a calibration sample. Others may calibrate less frequently than recommended by the device itself, ignoring calibration prompts.

While I understand how poor calibration practices happen, another part of me remains shocked. Our diabetes devices are no better or worse than how we use and maintain them. But people will do some pretty silly things sometimes, and healthcare professionals are not immune to outrageous behaviors like this. However, actions like these only undermine the usefulness of a glucose sensor. Poor calibration behaviors are seen in every age group using a CGM.

I wonder how many persons who complain about sensor inaccuracy also fall prey to poor calibration habits which might underlie their

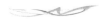

problem. As an experienced Sugar Surfer, I can attest that maintaining the accuracy of a sensor, relative to the meter, takes time and great attention to detail. I've found no short cuts to this. But the payoff for keeping your sensor properly calibrated at all times is huge. But even when the best calibration techniques are applied, sensors can still be at odds with a BG meter result. As discussed earlier, commercially available BG meters themselves are quite imperfect devices with significant potential for error. Sloppy technique on the part of the user can and will magnify meter error. A potential Sugar Surfer might be their own worst enemy (or ally) when it comes to maximizing sensor accuracy simply by how careful they collect BG calibration information with their meter. While some might give up and stop using the technology, I prefer to find ways to work through this and keep working to tighten up the calibration. But calibration is a constant, ongoing process and can't be ignored. This is where the core Surfing virtues of patience, consistency and resilience rule. Recommendations for optimal calibration will be discussed next.

A CGM can be no more accurate than the information used to calibrate it. The user must be able to properly collect and measure a blood sugar reading using a commercially available meter.

It's not the purpose of this book to recommend a brand of blood sugar meter; there are dozens available. Some have been proven to be more accurate than others under ideal testing conditions. Realize that meters are hardly used under "ideal" conditions by most patients over time. This is why user technique makes such a huge difference in the usefulness of the information obtained from any meter.

Remember, for many readers, a particular meter may not be covered by your health insurance provider. In that case you would have to purchase the desired meter and test strips on your own. Most people can't afford to do this or simply will accept whichever meter their health insurance covers. And based on the new reality that blood sugar meter devices are seen now as commodity items by insurers (where price trumps performance), it is likely you'll be required to change

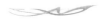

meters occasionally as generic BG meter providers negotiate lower cost bids to major health insurance plans or the government.

But regardless of the BG meter you use, always respect their inherent limitations and that they provide (at best) estimates of the blood sugar level from a tiny sample of blood obtained from the capillaries in your skin. Appreciate that your personal meter technique CAN be improved and serves to reduce the impact of the meter's limitations on your sensor accuracy.

Most sensors are unaware of the source of the BG reading entered into it and usually accepts what is entered without question. This opens up a huge door for error to creep in. The only exceptions to this principle were two of the earliest CGM's. One used a cable connection to the meter and the other CGM had an actual meter built into the receiver. Both of these designs have been discontinued.

At any point along the chain of collecting a BG reading from a finger stick blood sample, an incorrect reading is possible. If the sample site is not properly cleaned, then contaminants on the site could artificially raise or lower the reading. These contaminants include water, alcohol, food or drinks. If these mingle with the blood sample in any way, the sample is contaminated and at risk for giving an incorrect reading.

Currently approved meters also allow a certain amount of variability even under ideal circumstances. This is an ongoing area of controversy in diabetes care circles: the relative accuracy of a BG meter. To meet current 2013 ISO standards, the readings are allowed to vary from the actual reading (as measured by a highly accurate laboratory analyzer) by up to 20 mg/dL (1.1 mmol/L), 95% of the time. What might shock you is that in up to 5% of readings, the meter is "allowed" to be off by any amount, even hundreds.

Data from devices with this much variance are used to calibrate a CGM device. It's a challenge to maintain the best calibration habits you can to collect the most useful readings from your CGM device. It's also for these reasons that current devices are still more useful for the

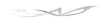

trending (directional) information they reveal than always being spot on with a meter reader. Although, if properly maintained and calibrated, they can be remarkably close.

Over the years since CGM has been introduced, calibration seems to be treated more as a nuisance than as a critical part of Sugar Surfing by both the patients who use them and by those who instruct on how to use these sensitive devices. When was the last time any diabetes professional reviewed how you actually perform a BG check or even watched you perform one directly? Probably never for most of us after the initial training. It's just assumed you know what you are doing. After years of watching children and teens measure BG levels at diabetes camps, I can attest there is a huge opportunity for improvement in the quality of BG data based on mastering a relatively simple set of actions.

To get the best results from your device, here are calibration tips that will improve the reliability of the data displayed by your receiver which in turn translates to your ability to more easily master the Sugar Surfing method.

1. Take your time and collect a quality BG sample.

This means cleaning the area to be sampled. The best approach is to use soap and warm water to get "junk" off the fingers (where most of us check) and get good blood flowing through the area. If you have to milk a blood sample after using your lancet, it could add additional fluid into the sample and dilute the reading. If you collect from a cold area, the blood might come out but the actual reading could be lower than the sugar in your main circulation since that capillary blood was pooling in your cold fingers. There is always a small difference between the sugar level in your arteries and veins compared to your capillaries (where we sample ourselves). So remember: clean, warm and dry is best.

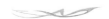

2. Calibrate your meter.

To make sure your sample is as accurate as possible, make sure your meter is also calibrated. This includes using control solution to test your strips for their own accuracy. It may not surprise you that the majority of BG meter users never use control solution(s) to check the accuracy of their test strips. Test strips that are old or damaged by moisture or heat will give incorrect results. Control solution is your best assurance that your BG checking kit is working properly.

3. If ever in doubt, perform a second (or even third) BG check if your BG reading seems at odds with how you feel, or if it's far away from the sensor readout.

If you are the user, the "how you feel" part is easier than if you're doing this to someone else. In that case, it's more about "how do they look" or "how are they acting" if you think the meter reading is not correct. This is one reason why some sensors require at least two readings at the start of a new sensor session. If I ever get results that don't match up with my personal sensations of high or low, I repeat another BG check to verify and check at another site. You might also check an extra BG and use the middle ground between the two values that are the closest together.

4. New sensor sessions are usually allowed to start after a couple hours of "warm up".

Experienced CGM users often note that the first day after placing a sensor can be more erratic than after the first day. Why? Most likely this is due to the fact that it takes time for a new sensor to reach its equilibrium with the body fluid it's measuring. Sensors are coated with a substance called a membrane which takes time to become fully 'wet'. Don't be surprised by erratic readings during the first 24 hours or so.

5. Medications.

While the list is not long, some medicines have been known to interfere with the CGM sensor apparatus. The most well-known has been acetaminophen, the active ingredient in Tylenol and other pain medications. I've personally noted polyethylene glycol to register on the sensor as glucose and confuse the device. The amount taken was large however (preparing for a colonoscopy). Most sensor companies deny there are many interfering substances aside from acetaminophen above (and that is just one company).

6. Be careful not to over-calibrate.

I often recheck BG after 4-6 hours with a new sensor, then another at 12-18 hours after insertion. The first day following a new sensor insertion is prone to be more erratic. It's wise to conduct a few more BG calibrations over and above the recommended minimum. In some cases entering too many calibrations each day might confuse the sensor software and trigger it to go offline for a while. If that happens, you can contact your CGM company's customer support line to make sure the system is not having other problems.

Hyper-calibration can be a common mistake made by some new sensor users. More doesn't mean better. Accuracy is not always improved with more calibrations. Don't remove a sensor when it stops reading. As I said, call the company help line as needed. In many cases, within 2 hours the sensor will be back online. It's good to perform a calibration after such a data gap.

7. Calibrate your sensor on a steady trend line.

As discussed earlier, modern sensors measure glucose in a different fluid space other than your actual blood sugar. There is a small amount of time that sugar takes to move from the blood and into the tissues (interstitial fluid, where sensors do their measuring). In order to get the best calibration, try to perform a calibration when your sensor shows a straight and relatively level trend line. In this case, it's best if you are

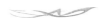

This page has been sponsored by: Lachlan John Robertson

seeing little change (no rapid shifting up or down) displayed on your sensor readout. This allows the device software to best pair your blood sugar to the interstitial sugar. One exception to this rule is "calibrating at the bend". I can often get a tighter calibration after I've administered an insulin dose (usually a meal or correction dose of rapid acting insulin) and "waiting for the bend" or inflection point along the trend line. This often happens about 15-25 minutes after the insulin dose. I've found this to be a good way to tighten up the match between the meter and the sensor. I consider this calibration technique to be advanced Sugar Surfing skill.

8. Calibrate in the range you want to be most accurate.

Most CGM devices will accept a calibration as high as 400 mg/dL. But don't think for one second that your device will be accurate at 85 mg/dL if the calibrations were mostly entered in higher ranges. I recommend correcting the high BG as you have been taught, then waiting until you get a sensor displaying a BG value in a range you prefer (and hopefully on a straight trend line) then recalibrate with your meter. Yes, it's an additional BG check but well worth the effort.

9. Re-calibrate when in range.

Whenever you deviate from your range, recalibrate when back in range. Sensor calibration is a finicky thing. If you have a BG spike or drop, you can calibrate to see how close to reality you (or your loved one) is, but when your readings seem to return back to your desired range, I suggest doing another calibration when back on a steady trend line. I call this phenomenon of distorting the accuracy of a calibrated sensor due to spikes and drops as "stretching the calibration". It's best dealt with by recalibrating when you get back to your home BG range.

10. Don't take short cuts.

This is where too many CGM users shoot themselves in the foot. As I mentioned earlier, I know diabetes health care professionals who personally use a CGM device (and who should know better) and skip

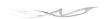

This page has been sponsored by: Kyle Smith

scheduled calibrations, simply re-enter the value of the sensor readout (don't want to be bothered to check a BG), or enter one single BG value twice at sensor start rather than two separately collected values. And this is in addition to the other calibration tips I've already discussed which they may not choose to perform. Just imagine what other users with less understanding about proper sensor use might do to shortcut this very important process.

Garbage in, garbage out. A CGM device is no better or worse than the person operating it. Before you condemn your sensor as "not accurate enough" take a closer look at how you treat it. The seduction of our diabetes technologies is in how they offer to make our lives "easier".

Getting a near continuous BG readout on a small screen can be a tremendous asset to our care. The trending information is invaluable for warning me to check for an impending low or high BG level which I confirm with my meter. And compared to the time, discomfort and overall effort it took me to collect any useful information about my blood sugar levels in the 1980's, these devices are truly miraculous. But diabetes care miracles usually have a price tag, in both time and money. I'm talking here about our time and attention to properly maintain it every day. The trade off is not having to spend hours later bringing blood sugar levels back in range and potentially missing out on some of life's greater pleasures in the meantime.

So why should anyone care how well calibrated their CGM device is? We all accept that their greatest value at this time is how they reveal trends even though they may not exactly pair up with a standard BG reading. Some of the reasons as to why this is the case have now been explained. In my case, I aim for near normal BG control. My target BG range is ambitious: 60 mg/dL to 140 mg/dL (3.3 – 7.8 mmol/L) with a target of 100 mg/dL (5.6 mmol/L). For me to be able to confidently keep my BG values in this range, I need my CGM device to be at its peak accuracy. I can only do that if I have maximum confidence in the readings on the display. Of course I combine these data with my own

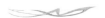

abilities to sense impending lows and highs, plus a constant sense of awareness of my situation: what I've recently done, what I'm doing now and what I plan to do soon. This actually doesn't take as much of my time as it sounds. But, since I believe that my diabetes control is always dynamic and "exists in the moment", this is my approach and why I can consistently maintain my A1C in the low 5% range with minimal risk of severe low blood sugar.

A pro surfer wouldn't hit the waves without first giving it a good wax job. You shouldn't expect good results without properly calibrating your CGM and meter.

Now, grab your board. It's time to surf!

Basic Concepts of Sugar Surfing

Chapter 7

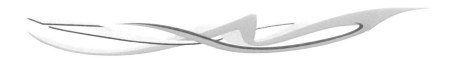

You've now reached the meat of the book. This chapter will take you step by step through all of the basic things you would do as a Sugar Surfer. This is the first step towards getting you started. To really be proficient and move on to the advanced concepts and maneuvers, you should become familiar and comfortable with the concepts in this chapter. You should have also read the instruction provided in the previous chapters. If you have 'cheated' and jumped ahead to this chapter without investing time in the earlier chapters, I encourage you to stop and start again from the beginning.

The primary concepts in this chapter are basal rate assessment, more on calibration, eating adjustments, setting your target ranges (sensor limits), glancing, micro-dosing and over-correction. I will close out the chapter with some "pearls" of wisdom related to Sugar Surfing.

Basal Rate/Dose Assessment

I'm always checking to make sure my basal insulin (whether it's coming from the basal rate programmed in my pump or a shot of long acting insulin like Lantus or Levemir) is working the way I want it to work. That usually means between meals and snacks, my BG trend line is fairly straight and not drifting too far up or too far down. A little drift happens even when things are going well and that is what nudging is all about. What I'm looking for is something that says I'm getting too much or too little basal insulin. If so, it means I'm going to drift pretty consistently up or down at a certain time of day without any obvious cause, like food, insulin, exercise or stress and makes trouble shooting unnecessarily difficult.

A medical explanation goes something like this. Sugar (glucose) is simply a cellular fuel. Tissues and organs depend on a steady stream of glucose as their primary source of energy. There is a constant process of entry and exit of sugar from the bloodstream every second of our lives. The amount of sugar dissolved into the liquid of our blood is the result of what comes into the bloodstream minus what is leaving. The body has many chemical systems that govern this process in both directions. Sugar Surfers need to understand some of the common ways these systems (or "tides") can shift, which can then affect the body's blood sugar levels. I will discuss these as they become important to know. One of those organs where keeping a steady flow of sugar is very important is the brain.

Our bodies must be able to provide a steady stream of sugar for not only the brain but also to other organs under a wide range of conditions or circumstances. From sleeping and total inactivity, to all-out physical exertion, competitive sports, stress, illness, and everything else in between, our body's need sugar. The liver and muscles are responsible for storing sugar for use between meals and for high intensity activities. The liver also produces new sugar from non-sugar substances inside the body (i.e. - fat and protein). The amount of insulin in the bloodstream, along with other body chemicals and hormones, controls

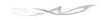

whether the liver takes sugar away from the bloodstream or releases sugar into it.

The body needs a small amount of insulin present in the blood at all times. This is necessary for keeping a steady stream of sugar going into the cells for energy and growth and to maintain the body's status quo. Muscles, fat, and the liver need insulin for these tissues and organs to increase their sugar intake. The brain doesn't need any insulin to take up sugar, but the brain needs enough sugar to operate properly. When sugar levels get too low (hypoglycemia), the brain starts to malfunction in many different ways. A non-diabetic pancreas (where the insulin is produced and released) has the ability to immediately stop releasing insulin under certain situations (low blood sugar and intense exercise being two of them). But persons taking insulin can't shut off insulin without some kind of effort (like withholding a scheduled insulin dose or stopping insulin delivery through a pump). And when they do, it still takes time an unnatural amount of time for the insulin already inside them to be washed out.

Insulin washout time depends on the type and amount of insulin being used. If an insulin pump is discontinued while only running the basal delivery, the duration of the insulin effect from the basal insulin usually lasts 1-2 hours before it's gone. If a dose of injected long acting insulin is stopped, it could be many more hours before the result would be noticed by changes in the BG level.

All people (with or without diabetes) need a tiny amount of active insulin in their bloodstream at all times. The purpose of this insulin is to keep their blood sugar levels in balance from minute to minute. This insulin is also responsible for fending off the development of ketones. It usually does not require much insulin effect to prevent ketones. In fact only one-tenth of the insulin needed to corral blood sugars into a normal range after eating a full meal is necessary to suppress the formation of large amounts of ketones. I discuss ketones later in the book. "Having balance" means getting yourself into a situation whereby sugar levels don't change dramatically from minute to minute.

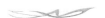

This insulin effect just quietly runs in the background. This is aptly called the "basal insulin" effect.

In diabetes management, the dose of basal insulin used is based on an expectation of a certain 'average' amount of activity and food being eaten. Basal insulin does not account for the separate doses of insulin that are used to help manage the change in sugar levels after eating food. Anything that upsets or changes that blood sugar expectation or balance could likely change the basal insulin need at that moment or even several hours into the future. This is another reason you should become comfortable with "ranges" of BG control. The forces that steer BG in and out of the bloodstream are numerous, in constant motion, and always interacting in some way.

The basis of testing the appropriateness of a basal insulin is whether its effect on glucose levels allow a generally stable BG trend in the absence of obvious forces known to raise or lower sugar levels. I liken this to having the steering properly aligned in an automobile. Otherwise, your vehicle would to one side or another while driving down a straight road. I wouldn't drive a car for long without this alignment nor would you.

In regards to all the forces that move blood sugar levels up or down, no two days are ever exactly the same. This is one reason blood sugar levels shift up and down even under the best of circumstances. If you are already on a pump and use multiple basal rates, what you will read next may challenge you. Always remember the 'goal' of a basal insulin rate: "To maintain BG trend stability in the absence of known forces that change BG (food, activity, stress)". The basal rate's job is NOT to change anything, but to maintain. Multiple insulin pump basal rates may be used to prevent anticipated changes in BG patterns, but they have no ability to react to unanticipated BG change no matter how many profiles you setup.

To get your basal insulin working well, aim to set up a basal profile that provides a fairly steady blood sugar tracing.

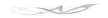

This page has been sponsored by: Kendall Tubbs

Morning Basal Checking and Monitoring

When I wake up each morning (or even if I wake up during the night), I usually reach for my sensor receiver to see where it "thinks" I am (my current CGM numerical readout). I also want to see where I've been and consider where I'm going. This is a really important thing to do and it only takes a

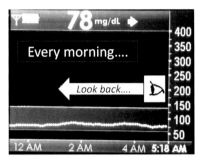

second. What I'm learning very quickly is how steady or straight my basal insulin (via injection or pump) kept my BG levels through the night, plus the effect of any foods I ate, exercise I performed, or strenuous activity undertaken from the night before. These three things are the primary drivers that influence my BG trend.

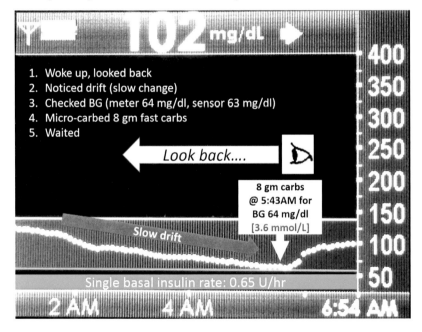

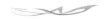

The minor amount of "wobble" that is sometimes seen on sensor tracings can be from laying on the sensor unit during sleep (pressure interference); from a very newly inserted sensor (not quite ready yet) or an aging sensor coming to the end of its useful life. When I mean new or old I mean how long the

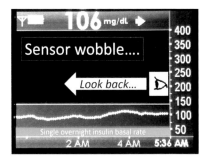

actual disposable sensor unit has been in place. A dying sensor transmitter battery may also be the cause of wobble. It's important to learn what is significant from what is just background noise on the sensor tracing. It takes time and patience to gain that experience.

What you will learn as you commit to performing this daily ritual is that even well managed BG levels will drift up and down a bit. And, even well managed and consistently in range basal rates are hard to predict. For whatever reasons, you will have days when your 'perfect' basal decides to go on a road trip and without even asking for permission. Your job as a Sugar Surfer is to expect the unexpected. Don't over-react to every sudden change you see at first. Taking a "wait and see" approach is always best at first. Expert surfers check out the beach geography, weather, water, and wildlife before ever jumping in with their board. Don't stress. Assess! Just think through the situation, use your training to correct the problem at hand and get on with your day.

As long as these basal tracings stay inside the upper and lower ranges I set for myself, I know my day is off to a great start. I'll show you how I manage the unexpected drifts later. As I say. "The only person with a straight line blood sugar is a dead person". Even non-diabetic people have BG patterns that move around, but a non-diabetic person's blood sugar generally stays somewhere between 60 and 200 mg/dL [3.3 - 11.1 mmol/L] all day every day. However most non-diabetic persons have BG values which travel in the lower half of this range most of the time.

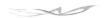

For emphasis, here's how you do it. Each morning when I wake up I look back to see how my blood sugars tracked while I slept. Things worked as I expected if I see a steady, fairly straight line trend. But if I don't see that relatively straight line in-range image, the next thing I do is think about what might have caused my line to drift or spike. My attitude is not how I went wrong, but how I can do better. Not judging harshly is how Sugar Surfers learn to improve their decision making skills. It also doesn't matter whether my basal insulin is delivered as an injection of long-acting insulin or from an insulin pump. I'm saying this more than once because these points are very important to remember.

When I first started using CGM I can tell you that having a steady trend line was not the case. However, over the years as I developed the Sugar Surfing method, my basal dose got optimally adjusted to meet my needs as I have described above. These days, my overnight trend line is usually 'straight-ish' or at least stays within my upper and lower limits.

If my morning basal tracings started to consistently trend upward or downward, I would suspect that my overnight basal insulin dose or pump settings might need adjusting and set out to do something about it. There are times when it trends up or down but I can often find a reasonable explanation. These might include such things as a slowly digesting meal (indicated by a slow rising BG), or lower carb intake or increased physical activity (indicated by a slow drop). These gradual drifts are not a good reason for changing the basal rate unless I plan on making a new habit out of the action I discovered to be causing the drift.

I started Sugar Surfing while using only injected insulin. That meant a single injection of long acting insulin served to meet my basal insulin needs. With careful attention to things other than insulin, I was able to maintain the same level of control on multi-dose insulin injections as I could with a pump (mid 5% A1C range). This implied that multiple basal rates might not contribute much to my overall control. I won't say my preferences need to be the same as others. We all need to find what

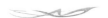

works on our own. Even when I pump, I run the fewest basal rates possible and usually just one rate for the entire day.

On those mornings when I happen to see a BG drift, I decide if I want to "nudge" the trend line. I nudge with either a micro-dose of insulin or a small amount of fast-acting carbs (see more about nudging and micro-dosing further on) depending on the direction of the drift. Contrary to what many do, I prefer to use the least number of basal rates. I use the same rate all day long and "nudge" the drifts as needed. If there were a clear and consistent pattern of up-drifting or down-drifting in my basal tracing over time (at least many days or a week or two), I would consider changing a basal rate segment if using a pump, or adjust the amount I injected if I was using long-acting insulin. Unless you've been taught how to make these changes on your own you would be wise to have this discussion with your doctor. It's beyond the scope of this book to explain the nuances of basal rate adjustments on pumps. What I can do is refer you to an excellent resource on the subject. Pick up a copy of "Pumping Insulin" by John Walsh for details.

Throughout-the-Day Basal Checking and Monitoring

Establishing that your morning basal BG tracing is in a range you want it is just part of the frequent basal monitoring you will do as a Sugar Surfer. This is something that should be done numerous times each day. I generally glance at my CGM 40 - 50 times a day. Information from my CGM glancing is integral to my ability to Sugar Surf. It's the driving force behind the "Plan - Do - Act - Check" cycle that Sugar Surfing teaches.

Actually, when I glance at my sensor readout, not only am I checking the BG number and the directional arrow but also the degree of pitch, the shape and potential inflection points in the trend line itself. If I suspect there is something to be done, I may look back over a longer time window to get a better idea of the trend line during the day. This quick trip down memory lane can be invaluable in helping me to recall how I got here and the result of choices I made earlier in the day. In

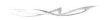

other cases, I may drill down and look at just the last few dots on the screen to see if the trend is starting to turn somehow. These abrupt changes in the trend line are called "inflection points" and they help me with my decision making. In contrast to downloading data from my CGM and analyzing patterns for hours, these quick glances have become second nature thanks to the invaluable insights gleaned about how my body works. Generalized diabetes training and education are one thing. Using these Sugar Surfing techniques to learn how your body works is priceless. I liken this approach to glancing at the dashboard as I'm driving my car. In a matter of seconds I get a quick status report of how my car is performing and if I need to be concerned about anything. It's a simple act with very powerful consequences for my "in the moment" diabetes control philosophy. So if you've not started doing it yet, just get into the habit of glancing at the sensor screen at least hourly while awake. Don't always feel the need to do anything at first, just be curious. I'll walk you through the rest.

As I said, when I'm glancing at the sensor screen, I'm usually looking at more than just the numerical value or the directional arrow. I'm also looking at the shape of the trend line over the past few hours or longer. It's my aim to wake up under 120 mg/dL (6.7 mmol/L) every day if possible. Ideally between 80-100 mg/dL (4.4 - 5.6 mmol/L). But I also know this is not always going to happen for reasons that may or may not be under my full control. It's important not to judge yourself for what you see. Even if your basal insulin settings were 'perfect', there will be some drift in the BG readings. No two days are ever alike, even if the insulin doses given are identical. That was discussed in False Idols, Chapter 5. Some of this drift (I also call it wobble) can be due to the imperfections of current CGM technology, but some of it is just human biology. As an endocrinologist, I've learned no system in the human body operates along a perfectly straight line, especially blood sugar levels. Everything shifts, it's only a matter of how much. Our bodies are designed to continually adapt to changing conditions and circumstances, we are not robots!

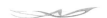

Look at this example of an experienced Sugar Surfer compared to a non-diabetic adult woman. It's hard to tell the difference between these two.

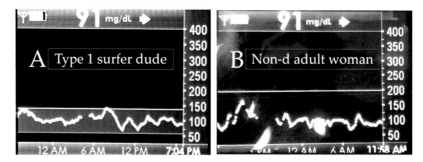

So, even when your basal insulin appears to have been working fine, there will still be those days where things spike or drift for reasons you can't control, discover, or understand. Don't despair. This happens to all of us, myself included. Sugar Surfing doesn't show you how to prevent all these random events, it teaches you how to responsibly act when these forces try to push your BG too far off course. It also allows you to discover those things you CAN change and keep from happening again, or occurring less often. Remember, Sugar Surfing puts you back in the driver's seat and diabetes in the back seat. That's a great feeling.

Get used to the practice of "looking back" each morning, as well as other times each day. It's a core Sugar Surfing principle not to be ignored! Eventually you will squeeze every bit of useful information out of a screen glance beyond just the number or arrow(s) displayed.

As a generalized observation, many people use too much basal insulin. When properly set, a basal insulin dose or pump delivery rate should not consistently raise or lower your blood sugar significantly by itself. This is true in the absence of significant stress, exercise, slowly digested food or lingering mealtime insulin. The accepted amount of BG drift allowed by a well set basal insulin is generally considered to be plus or minus 30 mg/dL [1.7 mmol/L] over time (that's a 60 mg/dL

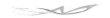

range [3.3 mmol/L]). Now think carefully about this: if your BG trend tracks steady over time, yet is well outside your chosen target range, this could actually indicate that your basal insulin is working properly. You just need to give yourself a bump of carbs or insulin to move that steady line into your target range.

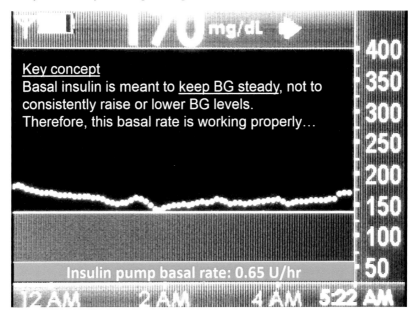

In this example, your basal insulin is simply keeping your BG tracing to where it was "moved" by a meal, a stressful event, an insulin dose, or some other BG raising or lowering "force". A properly set insulin basal rate is not supposed to bring you back to your target zone (up or down). That job is for a correction dose of insulin (to lower), carbs (to raise), activity (to lower), or if you are one of those folks who still make some of their own insulin, your own pancreas (to lower).

An object moving in space will travel in the same direction unless acted upon by an outside force. This is why spaceships have thrusters to maneuver them into new directions or precisely dock with other spacecraft. A well set basal rate behaves much like this example. Food, insulin, exercise and stress are some of the forces that can move the

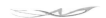

direction of the BG trend line that the basal rate is driving forward. Sugar Surfing aims to manipulate these forces to steer your own BG trend line.

I find that I can maintain equivalent basal insulin action whether I'm on a pump or using a long acting insulin by injection. So if you think Sugar Surfing requires an insulin pump, that's incorrect. There, I said it again.

Different Insulins. Different Result?

A note about the various short acting insulins out there. Unlike other people, I find no major differences between insulin lispro (trade name Humalog™), insulin aspart (trade name Novolog™) or insulin glulisine (trade name Apidra™) as far as Sugar Surfing goes. This is not to say there are not minor differences. Many will fervently believe one to be "faster" than another or have different duration of insulin action times. I will not debate that here. If you prefer a certain type of rapid acting insulin over another, I advise you to develop your Sugar Surfing technique around that formulation. Ocean surfers use different types of boards for different conditions but expert application of their knowledge of surfing is what matters most regardless of which board they might choose. Over time, when you reach Pro Sugar Surfer status, challenge yourself with a different brand of insulin and see how impactful it is. My guess is that even if you notice a difference it might seem insignificant when compared to the results you get by applying your hard earned Sugar Surfing skills. This simple act can be a very helpful experience in the event you cannot get your usual insulin and must substitute another.

As I said above, there are several brands of injected basal insulins now available. I advise you to choose one and stick with it. With time, practice, and careful observation of your BG trends, I believe a dedicated Sugar Surfer can tame any insulin preparation and make it work for them. Diabetes technology, including insulin, is no better or worse than the person using it.

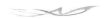

Ultimately, you must believe in yourself and your equipment. Tapping into your "Power Within" is a driving motivational force behind Sugar Surfing. In the end, success is determined by how much time and attention you invest into this process and less by whatever board you decided to surf that day.

Multiple Basal Rates

Many of the awesome BG tracings you see in this book were performed using my 10yr old insulin pump. It has all of the basic features I need. That said, people with T1D are faced with myriad and ever changing choice with regard to choosing their next insulin pump.

Although insulin pumps can have many basal rates programmed, I have rarely found more basal rates to be better than just a few, or one, when it comes to A1C levels. Making sure your basal insulin is set properly for your life situation is a basic skill that persons with diabetes should eventually master. Persons with advanced Sugar Surfing skills learn to manage the basal rate to offset highs and lows that might occur if settings remained unchanged, in the face changing situations. Learning when these changes are needed takes time and patience. The generous use of temporary basal rates is one step to determining if a more permanent change in your rate is necessary. I generally believe most patients using insulin pumps opt for more basal rates than they need. Simpler is usually better but exceptions abound.

It takes about 2 hours for the insulin effect to fully settle in following a pump basal rate change. That includes the changes you make manually as well as those that are programmed into your pump. Research that tracked the insulin effect of a basal rate changing from 0.5 to 1.0 to 2.0 Units/hour showed that the insulin effect itself "wobbled" even when the insulin was being given at a steady rate for hours. When the rate changed from 0.5 to 1.0 Units/hour, or from 1.0 to 2.0 Units/hour, it took about 2 hours until the new insulin effect took hold. Wobble in the insulin effect happened at any rate of insulin delivery. The pearls of wisdom here are that first it takes up to 2 hours to see the

full effect of a basal rate change when using an insulin pump. The second is that basal rates don't provide a steady insulin effect. This contributes to minor drifts in BG levels, but it's usually minimal. If you are changing a basal rate to pre-empt a trend (rise or fall), try to keep these timeframe dynamics in mind and make the rate changes far enough in advance of the expected effect you are seeking. This is the basic principle behind engine braking, which I discuss in Chapter 14, Surfing Rail to Rail.

But some persons already on an insulin pump may have many different basal rate segments programmed throughout the day. These extra rates might have been added due to a trend of high or low readings at a given time of the day or for a high morning BG or any of a number of reasons. The doctor or the patient might have made these changes. While I don't question whether the changes made a difference, I would ask whether the basal rate is being used for its intended reason...to maintain stable (notice that I didn't say "in-range") blood sugars in the absence of food, extreme activity or other stressors. The basal rate might be used more as a tool to manage poor eating or grazing behaviors or even omitted bolus insulin doses. Just ask yourself this simple question: "Will my multi-segment 24 hour basal rate profile allow me to have a fairly level trending BG pattern on more days of the week than if I were on fewer programmed rates?". If your answer is "no" or "maybe" then a change might be in order.

Other Factors to Consider

Overnight basal testing is easiest to check since there is usually less physical activity and no food or meal insulin to account for, overnight. But slow acting foods and late effects of prolonged exercise can confound even a properly set basal dose or rate. If there are carbohydrate snacks being consumed along with insulin doses, irregular sleep habits, illness, exercise, stress, or certain medications being used, then any or all of these could influence a basal BG trend overnight or at any other time. My point here is to always consider other suspects before laying blame on the basal rate and constantly

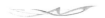

adding more rates. Sometimes simple is better.

During awake hours, the first step to test the effectiveness of a basal insulin is to withhold or delay a meal and avoid doing any things that are known to move sugar levels up or down. Actually, I tend to be very tolerant of drifting blood sugars and prefer to see a long standing trend pattern (up or down) before making a standing change in a pump basal rate or injected long acting insulin dose. It's why I've found a single 24 hour basal insulin or pump rate to work just fine for me. I realize that does not apply to everyone, but in general it helps to keep the total number of basal rates to the fewest needed, maybe 2 - 3 total. But we are all unique.

In some situations, doctors might prescribe running a high basal rate of insulin to offset the effect of excess snacking and overeating. This is most often used in hungry teens who are not interested in counting carbs or taking all their insulin boluses, but for some reason which I don't understand are still allowed to wear an insulin pump. Some diabetic persons who aim to lose weight yet eat what they wish will "ride the basal", rarely take any mealtime insulin and never take a correction dose or a meal bolus. Of course, BG control is poor in these situations. This type of diabetes "management" is not endorsed by me. Unfortunately, Sugar Surfing doesn't help folks who choose to live like this.

If you're missing scheduled insulin doses, not correcting out of range BG levels, and running a higher basal insulin to offset the effect of all this on your overall BG patterns ("riding the basal"), then you will need to commit to a paradigm shift in your diabetes management in order to Sugar Surf.

More on Calibration

In the morning when I wake up, there has been the maximum amount of time since any food was eaten or heavy exercise performed. Also, at this time of day my BG trend line is fairly straight (and hopefully in the BG range I aim for myself). I find this an ideal time to

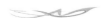

calibrate my sensor unit after washing my hands as described in Chapter 6, Waxing Your Board.

Warm hands mean better blood flow and a more realistic estimate of the BG in the rest of the body. For this reason, calibrating after a warm shower can be an excellent time to check blood sugar with your meter. This also takes into account my recommendation of calibrating your sensor on a steady trend line for the most accurate reading during the upcoming day.

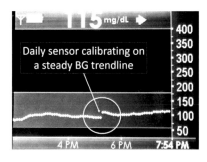

Calibrating before you start your day also allows you to calibrate the sensor before factors like food or stress can make a move on your nice, straight, in range BG trend. Regardless, calibrating in the early morning should be one of the first things you do each day.

Eating Adjustments

Based on what direction I see my trend line moving and the measured BG level indicated by my meter, I decide when it would be best to eat. It also instructs me as to what I should eat and how much. I've gotten to know the sugar raising impact or "profile" of several of my favorite food combinations through frequent practice and follow up observation. I use carb counting as a starting point, only. For bacon and eggs, or other low-carb containing meals, I may need no insulin (unless a correction was required before the meal). But for carb-heavy foods (cereals, breads, pancakes, Mexican food, pizza, chicken-fried steak-yum!), I must bring my A-game. It starts with a maneuver that I call "Waiting for the Bend".

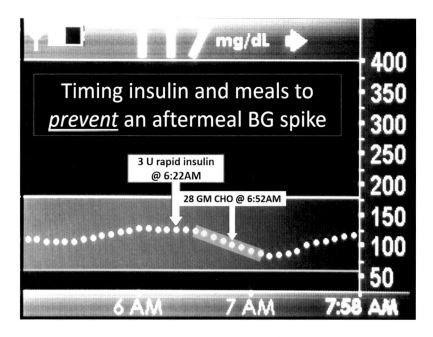

Injected insulin does not work instantly. The average accepted time from insulin injection to onset of action is roughly 20 minutes, but may differ slightly from person to person and time to time. Mealtime insulin is absorbed from the site of injection or infusion into tiny blood capillaries. Then it is taken through the blood to be delivered to all the cells which would use it. Insulin action is a process that has a beginning, a middle and an end. The medical terms are onset, peak and duration. Every type of injected insulin has these traits. A glucose sensor tracks changes in the level of sugar in the body tissues, which reflect BG levels in the blood. Remember, a sensor does not check insulin levels.

Once the level of sugar starts to fall, after a dose of rapid-acting insulin is given, its effect is indirectly "sensed" by the changing CGM readout.It's due to the ability to "see" (with glucose sensing) the time it takes for mealtime insulin to start working. This simple fact is what actually opens up a new world of opportunity for tightening up BG control. This concept is important to Sugar Surfing.

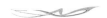

A signature benefit of a CGM device is its ability to allow its user to know the optimal time to eat a meal following the meal time insulin dose. It's very visual. Here I show when (and how much) insulin I injected for my anticipated breakfast. Waiting 20 - 30 minutes after injecting in this example, plus watching my trend line showed me the "window" (in light orange) when it would be best to eat my meal. These results speak for themselves.

Remember: at a hemoglobin A1C below 7.3%, it is estimated that two-thirds of the value is contributed by what happens to blood sugar levels after (NOT BEFORE) eating. This is one reason so many will struggle to break the sub-7% A1C barrier. By only checking pre-meal blood sugar levels you are helpless in your desire to manage diabetes. Knowing the after meal levels and correcting them when necessary with supplemental insulin, is the secret to attaining a sub 7% A1C. THIS is one secret to how I am always able to maintain a 5% - 6% A1C.

For many different reasons that are beyond the scope of this discussion, a meal-time insulin dose does not always start to work at the same time. I have numerous examples whereby it took over an hour for my meal dose to "bend" the curve in any way. In most of these cases the explanation was stress related. In another it was a pump catheter that was leaking (tunneling). But sometimes there is no obvious reason.

Waiting for the bend is simply a visual method to suggest or indicate that an insulin dose is actually reducing BG levels. As an experienced CGM user, I can often internally sense this process, and the sensor simply validates what I feel. I don't expect new Surfers to possess this ability at first. It comes with time and paying attention to internal sensations.

But waiting for the bend is only part of how I try to time my insulin and food. I've spent much of my time learning the pattern of the BG raising action of food products and meals I like to eat. My challenge is to match a meal to an insulin dose. Using standard insulin to carbohydrate ratios helps to a point. But, I also try to understand the

This page has been sponsored by: Janet Herman

speed at which each meal or food raises my BG level. To keep it simple, the terms slow, average and fast come to mind. Most of the time I'm not just eating a slow or fast carbohydrate food, but a combination of food types.

By studying my after meal BG profiles as they compare to an estimated insulin dose using my CGM, I use those results and experience to change how I make future attempts with the same food in a similar situation. How I do this will depend on the food and how it was prepared. In general, fried foods and whole grains are slow to convert to sugar, but as most people know, french fries and other fried carbs will raise BG quickly. It's beyond the scope of this book to profile all foods. Just understand that the foods you choose to eat will convert to sugar in the intestinal tract at different speeds. In fact, even the same food may have a slightly different glycemic profile the next time. This is due to factors like how the food was cooked and even how well it was chewed!

As I discussed in Chapter 5 – False Idols, I came to understand that all our diabetes care "constants", like insulin dosing formulas and carbohydrate counting, are riddled with variability. It's another reason Sugar Surfing makes so much good sense to me. I can't predict every force that will affect my BG levels and I never will. I can make elaborate plans based on my knowledge and experience, but I must always be prepared for the unexpected or seemingly random outcome. Diabetes care is both proactive and reactive and will forever be this way. Randomness, errors and omissions are everywhere in diabetes. Half of my work is in discovering it with my CGM and the rest is doing my best to counteract its effects. And, there is never any room for guilt in this process. Once again, this is what Sugar Surfing is all about: dynamic diabetes management 'in the moment'.

Newer ultra-rapid forms of insulin are already approved and under development. When these are widely available, it will require some changes in my Sugar Surfing moves, especially regarding timing these doses to eating. But, the basic Sugar Surfing concepts won't change. As

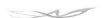

with every new technology introduced over the past 30 years, you can bet I'll be an early user and sure to test its limits.

Setting Your Target Range

It's important to set a "range" to try and keep your BG trends contained within.

When deciding on where to set your own targets, don't make it too hard at first. In other words, set higher and wider target ranges. The purpose is to first build confidence in your ability to steer your BG trend line within a range you're comfortable with. Just don't make it too narrow or too low. Aiming at 80-120 mg/dL (4.4 - 6.7 mmol/L) all the time is overdoing it. Non-diabetic people have wider BG ranges than that as described previously in this book. Alarm fatigue may result from setting overly ambitious BG targets; at least at first.

Alert thresholds for highs and lows, plus rates of BG rise and BG fall are adjustable by the Sugar Surfer. I routinely adjust my alert settings to suit the circumstances. For example, I set my low-high BG alerts to 140-180 mg/dL (7.8-10 mmol/L) for outdoor activities or doing heavy work. This is only temporary. Once I'm back to my usual routine I reset these thresholds back to my usual 60-140 mg/dL (3.3 - 7.8 mmol/L). If I'm treating a challenging high BG spike and know it might take a while to come down after taking a corrective dose of insulin, I may set the upper alert limit much higher for a few hours just to keep the alarm from going off too much. In these cases I'm fully aware I'm out of range and working to correct the matter. I don't need the additional distraction of frequent alarms going off. I just need to remember to reset it back to my usual settings when I'm back in my usual BG target zone.

Rate of BG change alerts are like having spotters on the beach scanning the horizon for potential trouble headed your way. If a sudden rise or fall in the BG trend occurs, these alerts are designed to inform you when your BG trend is dropping or rising at rates of either 2 mg/dL (0.1 mmol/L) per minute or 3 mg/dL (0.2 mmol/L) per minute. By getting an earlier 'heads up" to a rise or fall in progress, you have a

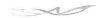

better chance to step in and blunt its effect if properly trained. If I am treating a very high BG level with insulin and waiting for the drop, I may set the fall rate alarm to tell me when my BG is falling even at the lower level of sensitivity (3 mg/dL [0.2 mmol/L] per minute). I will watch the fall until it approaches my target zone. I can turn these alerts on or off as needed. At night I may set my rate of change alarms to the highest level of sensitivity (2 mg/dL [0.1 mmol/L] per minute) to detect an early rise or fall. Remember, your sensor alerts are sentries and spotters for the Sugar Surfer. Learn to use them under different conditions to provide you the maximum assistance with the minimum of distraction. As time passes and your skills improve, you should gain confidence with BG and rate of change alerts. At that point you may consider setting tighter and lower low-high BG alert thresholds. But most of all, don't rush it.

Consider some point in the middle of your chosen range as your "pivot point". The value of this is discussed later. You can even just make it a "pivot range" rather than a specific number. It took me months to tighten my control ranges from where I started them. Remember… patience! Success is relative. If you start finding 250 mg/dL (13.9 mmol/L) or higher BG levels have become a thing of the past for you, no doubt you've moved in the right direction with your Sugar Surfing abilities. Sugar Surfing is a skill developed through a process, not a recipe or list of instructions.

Glancing

Glancing is something an experienced Sugar Surfer does all day long. You can't surf blindfolded. Glancing gives you the information you need to make adjustments throughout the day that help you stay within your chosen target range.

I intensify my glances as I navigate through obstacles like meals, activity, lows, or stress. I back off when I feel "ok" and might just look at the screen every 1 - 2 hours between meals. And, as I glance I'm also aware of the situation around me. I am aware of where my emergency

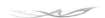

carbs are (in the car, in the bedroom, in my pocket). I will not be caught off guard, unprepared. Some might call me daring, but I'm not stupid. I want to stay at least one step ahead of my diabetes at all times. You can, too.

As non-active as my life may seem, it can become physically hectic sometimes. Of course some of you reading this book might be athletes or persons who spend a great deal of their time with busy work and travel schedules combined with erratic physical activity from day to day or even hour to hour. If that's not an indication to learn Sugar Surfing I don't know what is.

As I glance to see my BG direction, if I see a drifting high or low BG tide happening, I do a quick gut check. Is the trending high from late acting food, a basal rate drop I don't need anymore, stress about something in the office, or some combination of all three? After that short period of personal reflection (mere seconds), I choose whether I should watch the trend further, wait to see if it levels out, or step in and neutralize it with food, exercise, or insulin.

Even that decision requires some additional information. For example, ask yourself: "How soon will it be before I eat a snack or meal?". "Will I perhaps need some sugar energy for activity in the next hour?". If so, "Can a high blood sugar now be burned off later without insulin?". More serious issues could be: "Did I forget to bolus?". Or, "Is my insulin pump or my pump site not working properly?". Usually there is no shortage of questions you can ask yourself when you see a trend. There is usually a short list of common reasons that can help you explain why an insulin and meal event didn't work out as expected but sometimes not.

You will eventually create your own personal list of possible suspects, but please don't let guilt or fear have a spot in your mental situation room. Your glucose tracing possesses no morality. It's a visual representation of a biological process. Nothing more, nothing less. Fear and guilt are like dense seaweed to an ocean surfer. Don't let it pull you

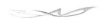

down. Rid yourself of these emotions as often as you can. Don't give diabetes any more dominance over you than it should. Respect it, yes. Fear it or feel guilt over it? Absolutely not!

Micro-Dosing and Micro-Carbing

Many of us treat our lows with carbs (fast or otherwise) until we feel better. Sadly, that usually means we over treat ourselves and will later rocket up to a BG over 200-300 mg/dL (11.1 – 16.7 mmol/L) and start the blood sugar roller coaster. Over treating lows is very easy to do when you or a loved one are in the grips of a severe, symptomatic low BG. For many people it seems to be the smartest, or the only thing to do, if not a treat in some cases. A time when it seems fair that you should be able to eat any sweet food or drink you wish and without guilt from the diabetes police. I don't fault anyone for doing this, as I have been just as prone to do it myself. Just be aware that it's a choice… your choice!

I first developed personal knowledge of my BG response to smaller carb doses based on taking small carb amounts at relatively higher straight line trends just to get a range of responses. I call this "nudging" and it usually is faster to raise a trending low BG than it is to raise a slow trending high BG. Plus it helps to make sure a clear and definite trend is happening and you confirm it with a BG check.

When you wonder why your BG went ballistic after consuming 1 or 2 juice bottles it might just be that you over treated the situation. Now... if your insulin is peaking and you are not on a level trend, then such larger carb dosing is certainly understandable and might be necessary. If you don't have a CGM showing you the trending direction or you are unwilling or unable to check every 15 minutes with your meter, then the Rule of 15 must be followed even if it results in a BG overshoot afterwards. It's always better to be safe than sorry… or worse.

For those of us who have been "rescued" from a severe low BG with oral carbs like honey, juice, glucose gel, or with a glucagon injection, overcorrection with carbs is common and sometimes necessary.

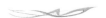

This page has been sponsored by: James G. Alexander

Remember, there is a lag time between the current CGM display and your actual BG during this time. The people treating your low BG will most likely continue to "shovel in" the carbs until the symptoms start to resolve. Once your BG is back up, use correction doses and Sugar Surfing techniques to get yourself back on track while being patient as you steadily move back down into range. Learn from the event and keep moving forward.

Micro-dosing and micro-carbing involve ranges of insulin and carbs rather than exact amounts. My definition of micro-carbing is taking from four to twelve grams of carb to bump up or nudge a falling BG. One standard glucose tab contains four grams of carb. Micro-bolusing is the injection of one (1) to four (4) units of insulin to bump down a rising BG. But these definitions only apply to me. Your micro-dosing tools will be specific to you and must be discovered by you. Here's how.

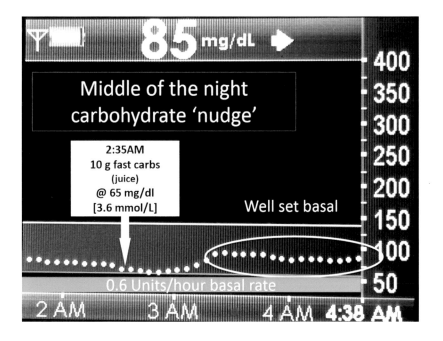

Safe experimentation is at the heart of Sugar Surfing. Whenever doing a personal Sugar Surfing experiment, it must be properly planned, carefully monitored and followed up with appropriate actions. Learning how to nudge (e.g. - micro-dose) is a great example of finding your own unique range of responses. For those of you just getting started, I use the following example of how I use this skill.

Learning how to micro-dose depends on having a well set basal insulin dose or rate via an insulin pump. This was discussed in detail earlier in this chapter. Much like a tugboat nudging a large ship into port, smaller doses of insulin and carbs can nudge a BG trend line that is properly glanced at over time.

What I'm about to say next may sound odd, but it's how to learn micro-dosing. First, find a stretch of time where you have a nearly straight line BG trend with minimal to no drift up or down. While on this straight line trend, eat a measured amount of fast-acting carbs (i.e.: a 4 gram glucose tab or 5 grams of fruit juice). Just make sure you are trending straight, not near a high or low alert threshold, and eat only a small amount of carbs (4-10 grams).

Then, wait and watch the trend line over the next 30-45 minutes as you go about your routine. Please note that the "routine" should not include any strenuous activity or anything else that you already know might affect the BG outcome.

What you are doing is carb calibrating; seeing what a small amount of carbs will do to your BG trend line. Make a note of the size of the shift, and make sure you watch it long enough. In other words, give it sufficient time until the trend line levels out. Be patient.

Once you've done your first successful micro-carb experiment, get ready to do many, many more. Like any other skill, it takes repetitive acts before proficiency is achieved. Confidence follows. It took me weeks to get comfortable with what 4 grams of glucose would do for a steady trend line. Generally it raises my BG about 12-15 mg/dL [+/- 1 mmol/L] from the baseline. I weigh 165 pounds (12 stone) so this

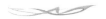

response would be very different in someone smaller or heavier, even of a different age and gender, and with a different duration of diabetes. The message here is that you must chart (and remember) your own unique responses to small carb amounts. And you should think in ranges of BG response rather than exact number difference. Mastering the art of micro-carbing takes time, but it is time well spent.

Micro-carbing should not be used when one is in the grips of a mealtime insulin dose or large correction dose of insulin which is dropping the BG level. This is not a time where a subtle response to an impending low will be very helpful.

In these cases treat by the accepted "Rule of 15" and watch BG carefully using your sensor, verified with your BG meter. I will discuss duration of insulin action and stacking insulin in greater detail later, but micro-carbing is not helpful while a mealtime or large high BG correction insulin dose is still working.

This period of time depends on the amount of the dose and the time since that dose was taken. If a combination bolus was being used via pump (where the continuous rate of insulin delivery is raised for a user-defined period of time), then micro-carbing may also be under effective and larger carb amounts would be needed to counteract a low trending BG level. Extreme situations will be discussed in Chapter 14, Surfing Rail to Rail.

To summarize micro-carbing, it's best done when the only insulin working is the basal. Practice this skill under safe conditions and not when your BG is near the upper or lower alert thresholds (at least at first). Do this many, many, times until you know the range of responses you will get. Always have corrective insulin available if you overdo it and correct a resulting high BG as you have been previously taught to do.

Micro-dosing of insulin is the complement to micro-carbing. Learning how to micro-dose might seem scarier than with micro-

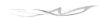

carbing because it involves taking insulin in a way we are not taught to do. But it can be done safely.

As I discussed in Chapter 5, mathematical formulas used to determine how much 1 unit of insulin lowers an out of range blood sugar value provide at best only a rough estimate in most cases. But CGM technology now makes it possible to refine these estimates by revealing the actual BG results of an insulin dose as it happens in real time. Once there was a method to safely administer small doses of rapid acting insulin and then track the result, micro-dosing was born. There is now a viable method to make minor or modest changes in the BG trend line, aimed at steering the BG trend line. That's Sugar Surfing!

More importantly, these micro-doses would be taken at times when blood sugar is already in range. Never before has that act been considered practical. Blood sugar control can now be fine-tuned throughout the day.

When setting up your experiment, it's also ideal to be trending along a BG value in the upper half of your target range. This might be above 120 mg/dL (6.7 mmol/L) for starters. Start even higher if the surfer is a child. Once the situation is safely setup as outlined above, take the lowest dose of insulin that your assigned insulin correction ratio allows. For example, if your ratio is 1 unit for every 50 mg/dL (2.8 mmol/L) over your target BG, then start with 1 unit if your trending BG is 150 mg/dL (8.3 mmol/L). If you want to be ultra-safe, then give half of that amount. Since the reduction would put you at 100 mg/dL (5.6 mmol/L) in two hours based on the formula, then wait and see what happens by glancing at the CGM over the next 1-2 hours. If this is being used in someone who is very sensitive to insulin, then consider reducing the starting dose by 75% or more.

Remember that micro-bolusing is best tested under non-extreme circumstances. Avoid strenuous activity that might magnify the effect of the insulin. Don't try to learn this technique when sick or taking medicines known to affect or raise BG levels, like oral steroids. Also

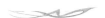

don't do this within 2 - 3 hours of another rapid acting insulin dose. Remember to check your BG when you take the dose and use the information to calibrate the sensor.

After the effect of the dose is seen on the screen in 1 - 3 hours, then recheck BG to verify the change and use that information as a calibration point for the sensor. But always keep in mind that there are unseen variables constantly at work. This is not science, just a form of diabetes art.

If you see a result, make a note of the change in BG level from the first to the second reading. Note the readings on the sensor as well. Make sure both results match up with each other fairly well. Rarely will they be spot on with each other, but it's the amount of change that matters most.

Once you've done a few of these, they get easier. In fact you will find that practicing this is more about being opportunistic than planning these sessions in advance. Focus on practicing with the range of insulin micro-doses that usually can move your BG 20 - 40 mg/dL (1-2.2 mmol/L) under steady trending conditions.

Once you get good at doing this during the week, just keep on practicing: for weeks to months.

In fact, you never really stop practicing this skill. Like waking up each morning and looking back at the basal trend line, micro-dosing is a constant consideration that you never stop thinking about. A working pancreas is always ready to respond to an out of range BG trend. Why should your approach be any less? That's how you start micro-bolusing insulin.

This page has been sponsored by: Indiana Dormer

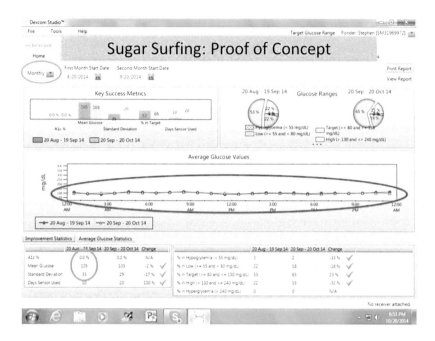

As you develop competence with insulin micro-bolusing, consider lowering your action threshold. I started off at 150 mg/dL (8.3 mmol/L). Once I felt ready, I moved to 120 mg/dL (6.7 mmol/L) and I now aim at 100 mg/dL (5.6 mmol/L) most of the time, depending on the situation or what I'm doing. However, I plan to run higher when involved in physical activity. Here is a readout showing a typical month of 24 hour sensor data showing how effective this strategy can be. I feel it's a good example of Sugar Surfing.

Once I cross my high BG alert threshold, I decide how to best "turn" the trend. I will see how long the trend has been moving and at what angle it seems to be changing. I can liken the rate of change to the physical concept of momentum. Slower trends, I call them drifts, are easier to turn than rapid shifts, which I call flux (you might prefer spikes). Here is an image of what I call flux and drift.

Turning a drift or spike might just be done with an insulin dose, but I might add exercise to it and reduce the insulin or eliminate it altogether depending on the situation. But as long as I continue to glance often at my trend line, I can navigate through whatever choice I make to turn the trend. At

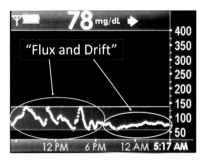

first, I used simple actions (insulin only, no activity or exercise, no additional insulin over the basic high BG correction dose calculation) and monitored their effects via my CGM receiver display and verified by meter BG. Only later did I start to blend them together (a lower insulin dose combined with a modest amount of exercise like a run or brisk walk). In EVERY case I monitored my progress by frequent glances at my sensor readout. This is one example of how Sugar Surfing is different than just a person using CGM.

What micro-dosing carbs and insulin taught me was that I could now, with the aid of a CGM device, fine tune or steer my BG trend line if I had the patience, preparation and practice to learn how to do so.

Caution: Over-correction!

Most persons with type 1 diabetes have over treated a low blood sugar level at one time or another. The usual approach to teaching and treating low blood sugar is based on the "Rule of 15". This rule states that a low blood sugar is treated by 15 grams of fast acting carbohydrates by mouth. Blood sugar is then rechecked in 15 minutes. Repeat as necessary until you see improvement based on BG checks. Very easy, very simple... and highly variable in its response. Even so, in most cases it raises BG quite a bit. But the rule is designed to over treat, based on the common sense principle of "better safe than sorry". But in the era of Sugar Surfing, we can now do better.

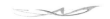

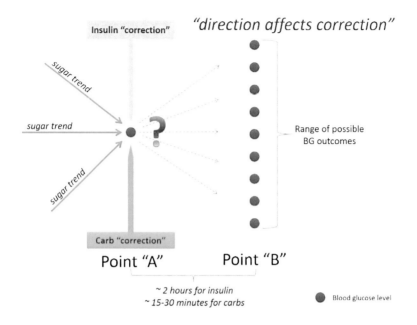

Sugar Surfing offers a better option. The Rule of 15 is about as subtle as a sledgehammer for younger persons, and may barely effect a low sugar level in an older teen, adult, or a larger persons. But it's more than just the blood sugar level itself that plays a role regarding what happens next. For example, if the blood sugar is trending down or up, this could seriously affect the blood sugar response to 15 grams of fast acting carbs or glucose tabs. Problem is, until recently we lacked the ability to see these blood sugar trends without lots of BG checks back to back. CGM has opened our eyes to the fact that "direction affects correction" as I teach.

Here's a simple example. It shows the effect of a small dose of carbs (about 10 grams) on a "steady state low" blood sugar.

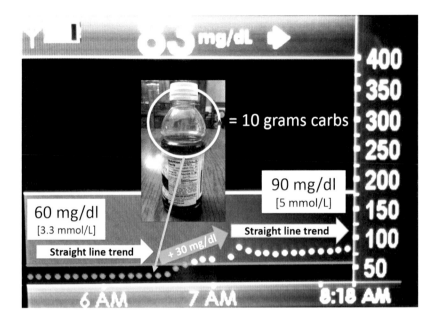

My CGM was reading slightly under its actual level based on my meter. The sensor said "LOW" but I was in the low 60 mg/dL (3.3 mmol/L) range and was not very symptomatic based on a meter BG check. I was not dropping or increasing as you can see on the left. So... I consumed a small amount of carbs which contained a total of 10 grams of carb). Then I waited for what I KNEW would happen next: a 20 - 30 mg/dL (1-1.6 mmol/L) rise in sugar levels as you see in the middle of the graph. NO over-treatment of a low.

The image on the next page is an example of a 'low' treated at a diabetes camp. At camp, we have traditionally treated any BG under 120 mg/dL (6.7 mmol/L) at midnight to prevent a low due to high activity during the day. Clearly the BG was raised, but by a much larger amount than expected. Because of this we decided to review policy and implement small carb doses in the future in CGM enabled campers. Of course, we raised his BG but we over-treated it too!

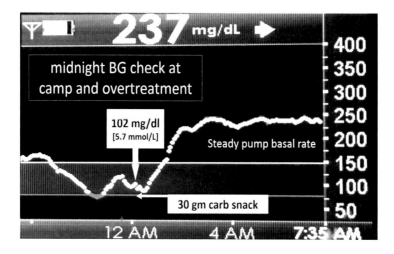

The Three Virtues

At this point in the chapter, I would like to remind you of the three virtues of Sugar Surfing: patience, consistency and resilience. To perform Sugar Surfing methods well, work to include these three attitudes in your mental toolkit when approaching any diabetes challenge you encounter.

Patience is my hardest virtue to maintain. I want insulin and food to work faster than they really do. But waiting for a turn or bend after a micro-dose or a meal dose of insulin is a reward unto itself. Also, it does take time for a proper dose of fast acting carbs to slow down and reverse a dropping BG trend. Many of us, myself included, may over-treat a trending low instead of waiting for the tracing to flatten out from its downward trend. Hint: try to treat a trending low at a higher point than the low threshold alert setting on your CGM. For example, if your low alert is programmed at 80 mg/dL (4.4 mmol/L) and you see a downward trend crossing 90 mg/dL (5.0 mmol/L), treat with your "proper" amount of carbs and wait to see how long the trend line will take to level off. Remember, the lines act as they have some amount of momentum behind them. Taking that to an extreme, if you see double arrows down, you would choose to treat at an even higher threshold, ideally after checking a meter BG to verify the drop. You must be

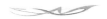

patient in mapping out your unique range of responses.

Consistency is important for the simple reason you want to have a standard or somewhat reliable way of doing certain things. I have learned through consistency and lots of practice just how much 4 grams and 10 grams of fast acting carbs will affect my BG trends. I have learned how much 1, 2, 3, 4, 5 and up to 8 units will lower my BG by practicing and watching the results and remembering them. I also know that these results differ depending on how high my blood sugar is when I correct, and how fast the drop is. This is illustrated in these two slides showing how I "take the drop" at 140 mg/dL (7.8 mmol/L) or 180 mg/dL (10 mmol/L) with 3 or 6 units rapid-acting insulin, respectively. Both will lower my BG to a tight range and rarely overshoot. But if I do, I can correct it.

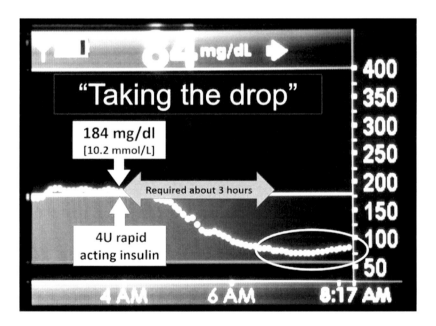

Resilience is the third Sugar Surfing virtue. I made mistakes in both directions in learning how to pivot, plus many other parts of developing how to Sugar Surf. I realized that static formulas were only

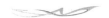

a starting point to figure how much insulin to use to treat an out of range BG, or haw many carbs were needed to treat a low BG.

I also had to remember that the direction my BG was moving would affect how well my choice of insulin dose amount or grams of carbs would best work. Through careful trial and error experimentation (with very careful watching of the CGM screen after each decision), I was able to better estimate what I needed.

What I found was that if I had given up after the first few tries, this book would never have been written, at least not by me.

To master Sugar Surfing you must be willing to try, do, fail and learn, then repeat the cycle all over again. That's how we get better at something. But there is no way all the answers can be served up to you on a silver platter. You must learn them for yourselves.

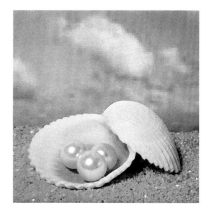

Well that's a lot of information to digest. I will try to boil this down to some helpful Sugar Surfing pearls of wisdom. An accomplished Sugar Surfer uses these pearls every day. Over time, with much practice, these will become second nature to you, too!

1. Assess basal insulin action.

Wake up and check your overnight trend (look back). Is it steady, in range or out of range? Calibrate sensor with a meter check (if steady trend and before the day can affect your BG). If needed, troubleshoot. Nudge by micro-dosing carbs or insulin if out of range. Use correction doses as needed to correct spikes and treat severe low BG with fast acting carbs.

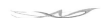

2. Calibrate your sensor and meter regularly.

CGM and meter readings are the bedrock of Sugar Surfing. Accurate data is essential to all Sugar Surfing decisions and actions. If you skip this step, you are surfing blind. Set wider and higher BG alert thresholds at first. As your CGM competency evolves into CGM proficiency, lower and tighten these ranges to best meet your needs. Feel free to change them 'in the moment' to adjust for special circumstances.

3. Time insulin doses ahead of meals

Ask yourself what you will eat, when will you eat, and what else is going on that might affect your BG. This is called "situational awareness". Make sure you know what your BG is when you take that pre-meal dose. BG steady and above 60 mg/dL (3.3 mmol/L)? Bolus and wait 20 minutes. BG dropping already or having a low carb or slow carb meal? Consider dosing later or use a combo/extended insulin bolus. "Wait for the Bend" before you eat. If you are really hungry, eat the fat/protein first and eat carbs after the bend.

4. Glance at the CGM often

Look at your CGM display MANY times each day (40 – 50 times/day is NOT too often). Glancing gives you the info you need to make the adjustments throughout the day. Be mindful of your Situational Awareness and Targets. Slow down! Spend 20 seconds every time you check your blood sugar or before you commit to a blood sugar affecting event. By contemplating where you've been, where you are now and what you are about to do, you will make better decisions. As you progress with your surfing, the time needed to arrive at your next move will decrease. Increase your glances as you navigate through obstacles like meals, activity, lows, or stress. You can back off when you are/feel steady.

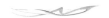

This page has been sponsored by: Etienne Reyes

5. Watch trend lines

When you first wake up, assess your basal insulin's effectiveness. After eating meals or snacks, glance to pick up unexpected spikes or drops in BG. Check BG 2 - 3 hours after eating and correct an out-of-range reading back to your pivot point. Remember to adjust with carbs or insulin based on other factors (exercise or stress). Learn to adjust BG rate of rise or fall to best suit the circumstances. These are spotters that 'have your back' when you are not watching the CGM readout like during sleep or when other activities require your close attention.

6. Use micro-dosing to manage blood glucose drift

Nudge slowly drifting BG levels if the drift is steady and be patient over at least 30 minutes to an hour. Pre-empt rapidly rising or dropping BG using insulin or fast acting carbs. Experiment with micro-dosing carbs or insulin over a stable BG tracing to learn the effect of these adjustments on you. Do this several times so you can learn YOUR body's trends. While you are new to this process and learning, keep a journal of how meals, snacks, insulin doses, micro-dosing and activity personally affects your BG. Looking for patterns or consistency (or lack thereof) requires that you repeat the same process. Mastering the art of micro-dosing takes time and it is time well spent.

7. Don't be afraid to take action

Review your data and make a decision. Follow that with action. Assess the result of that action in the appropriate time frame. If your assessment indicates another action (or no further action) is immediately needed, act accordingly. Plan, Do, Act, Check. Repeat this cycle. This is a "closed loop" system that you repeat many times each day. Don't be afraid to make errors. If a decision you made does not turn out as expected, do a deep dive to find out why, and learn from it. Use that knowledge when making future decisions.

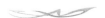

There you have it. The fact that you are reading this book proves that you're already taking action to educate yourself and/or reinforce your beliefs about having better BG results and live a more normal life. Good for you! Now you have to act again by making sure you put all of these tools into practice.

Feeling like you don't have 20 seconds to assess a situation? Nonsense. And if you took an action that turned out to not be the best choice, at least you made a choice. It's my belief that simply being more engaged in the moment will make your life, and your diabetes control, better.

Sugar Surfing & Children

Chapter 8

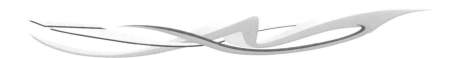

KIDS CAN SURF, TOO!

Much of the material in this book might be considered strictly for adults. But Sugar Surfing principles can benefit persons with diabetes of all ages. I know families of toddlers, pre-teens and teens who routinely apply some or all of these concepts in their day to day approach to diabetes care.

It is not my expectation that all the Surfing tools described in this book can be used in children. Some can, some can't. And even the ones that can be helpful in children may not be used all the time for many different reasons related to circumstances in the moment. But even if you apply just a fraction of these methods, I believe you will see improvement over time. The techniques also take time and practice to develop a sense of confidence and mastery in their use. So be persistent, use these skills when you can, and don't give up. Children cannot become effective Sugar Surfers without well involved parents supporting them, period.

Here is an example sent to me from a mom in Canada and another from America. I'm fond of the term the girl adopted to describe her in-range trend patterns as "Dr. Ponder Lines".

"Dr. Ponder lines" in a 7 year old Canadian Sugar Surfer

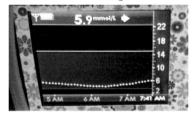

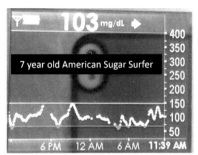

7 year old American Sugar Surfer

By necessity the Sugar Surfing family works as a team. This forms a foundation of tighter blood sugar control as the child grows up and when I say 'child' I mean up to at least age 16. It also allows the family to stay engaged in care longer.

Basic Sugar Surfing principles are the same no matter your age:

a) Look at your trend line often.

b) Maintain and calibrate the sensor properly.

c) Always keep your eye on how your basal insulin is working to keep you on a steady trend line.

d) Balance the time when you take insulin and eat using the sensor as a guide.

e) Learn how to micro-dose carbs and how to micro-bolus rapid-acting insulin safely.

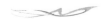

This page has been sponsored by: Emma Duncan

Issues related to readiness to wear or use a sensor.

Are most kids really willing to do this? Will he/she see its benefits in the same way mom and dad do? Many children view their diabetes differently than their parents. To them diabetes is just a lot of finger pokes and insulin shots, feeling like all you get told anymore is what you can and can't eat or do, feeling weird and cranky when low sugars happen, and feeling thirsty, crabby, and crazy active when high sugars happen.

So asking a kid to wear a sensor when they might already be wearing an insulin pump might seem like the straw that broke the camel's back. Plus young children have fewer attachment sites for applying a sensor every week and a new pump site every 2 - 3 days. Younger kids might also cry and fuss when the sensor is being inserted. Although, there are very effective prescription numbing creams that can be placed on the skin an hour or so before putting on sensor that can make it pretty pain-free. You will need to ask your doctor for those. Some docs don't approve while others do.

Some kids (and grownups) don't want to have anything attached to them, period. It may take some time for them to get over this idea, if ever. When I hear this I must respect those wishes and I discourage anyone to compel a child or teen over age 7 to wear such a device. It could cause more harm than good. In these situations, it might be possible to wear a sensor on a trial basis. Afterwards, the original fears harbored by the child might pass. Or it might affirm their decision to not use this technology. Parents should then put the issue aside and wait a while. As the child matures, attitudes might change.

Early studies with sensors and children found benefits to BG control only in those willing to wear them often enough, typically at least 85% of the time. Early generation sensors were also larger and more difficult to wear and maintain. Many children and some adults found the length and diameter of early generation sensor probes both imposing and painful to insert. Since many early sensor users were already wearing

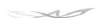

insulin pumps, a certain amount of technology fatigue occurred. This lowered the enthusiasm in some children and teens that had to wear "one more thing" to care for their diabetes. Plus, since the primary benefit of a glucose sensor (information) is quite different than an insulin pump (convenience), children were not as appreciative of their value. Today's sensors have become smaller and easier to insert. As mentioned above, the proper use of prescription topical anesthetic creams, or even the application of an ice pack to the sensor site to numb the skin, can lessen any discomfort of sensor insertion.

Asking (or allowing) your child or teen to take a sensor vacation can be a good thing once you've seen improved control and diabetes care skills as a result of continuous use. Other reasons to go sensor free might be when on vacations or if involved with high impact sports like football. Parents might be the most nervous about a sensor break, since they may have become accustomed to always having BG data available. It could almost be like a withdrawal state for some heavily invested moms and dads.

Some children may view CGM as a method for parents to oversee all their actions. This attitude might be more acute if the family uses a real time data transfer device to share CGM data with other family members. While BG data sharing is a powerful tool, kids may also perceive it as an invasion of their personal privacy and passively or actively resist wearing them or become subversive in manipulating blood sugar data. Parents should consider why they are making this choice and include the child or teen in the decision. In many cases sensors provide a level of comfort to the family in detecting episodes of low blood sugar, especially when the child sleeps. Very young children cannot object to a sensor due to their age. They may not tolerate wearing the device and may pull it off or get intensely fearful when it's time to insert a new sensor. This fear generally fades with time. Better site preparation and insertion technique will help.

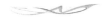

This page has been sponsored by: Durham Family

Parents: check your attitudes first

I advise parents of children with diabetes that if they treat their child as handicapped by their condition, after a while they may start acting that way. There is a psychological phenomenon known as learned helplessness and it plays a huge role in how people with diabetes and their loved ones manage the disease. Parents may see their child with diabetes as especially vulnerable and in constant need of their help. While this is part of the natural process of being a parent, the degree to which this attitude is taken becomes smothering both to parent and child. Through interactions with health care providers, social media, close friends and family members, parents and persons with diabetes "learn" that they have a serious medical condition which is unpredictable, will impact their lives in many different ways (mostly bad), and can at times even be deadly. This point of view creates a mental shell that many parents and persons with diabetes retreat into, refusing to consider diabetes care approaches that might allow greater independence or flexibility.

I advise all my patients with diabetes that my first and foremost goal for them is to live a normal life. It's not about numbers. A sensor can help some children to achieve that goal as it has for me, but it's the attitude of the family that best defines the direction of the child's life with diabetes and how they will incorporate it into their lives.

Getting involved and staying involved

In spite of how often they might look at their cell phones each day, older children and teens typically don't glance at their CGM readouts nearly as often. This is largely because they don't know how to interpret what they are seeing beyond the number or arrow on the screen. The blood sugar dot line is the most valuable piece of information displayed because it reveals a trend that the child or teen should pay attention to. Sensor alert alarms notify the child only if they're paying attention to the sounds or vibrations of the receiver unit. But like adults, they can get distracted or simply ignore alerts when

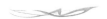

they occur. CGM technology has already progressed into the era of transmitting data to a cell phones and watches and exercise bracelets in addition to the standard receiving device. While it is possible that teen CGM users might become more engaged with their data as a side effect of their collective obsession with their phones and other tech gadgets, each child will determine for themselves how much interaction they will undertake.

Every child with diabetes is unique with their own set of likes, dislikes and personal goals. Since these goals are often not related to how they manage their diabetes or share self-care responsibilities with their parents or caregivers, this will always be a source of ongoing distress for parents. You can place a sensor on a kid, but you can't make them care. In older children and teens, make sure the sensor is being purchased for the kid, not for the parents.

Glancing

I glance at my sensor up to 40 - 50 times a day although the average CGM user looks up to 20 times daily. The action itself only takes seconds and can be done discreetly or while doing other tasks. Glancing is important at all ages since Sugar Surfing is about being aware of the situation at hand and managing the BG trend line in the moment. If a trend line looks concerning, such as a steadily downward or rapidly rising trend line, I'll stop and give it and the situation more thoughtful consideration and reflection. Ideally, you should have been taught to do this action with every standard BG check from your meter, but many have never been taught this skill. You might be of the belief that these data are mostly for someone else to study, right? Just the opposite. These BG trends are for you to put to work immediately to make better informed self-care choices. The child or teen needs to be taught what patterns need attention sooner than others and to alert the parent (if needed) so definitive action can be taken before a poor result occurs (severe high or low BG). If your child can master the dynamic rapid-fire visual action of handheld video games, Sugar Surfing may seem like a slow motion walk in the park to most children and teens with diabetes.

Relating CGM to teens

Actually, when I explain Sugar Surfing to children and teens, I typically conjure up the idea of a video game. After all, a sensor receiver readout could be likened to a gaming console. But I go on to explain that the CGM user is the avatar. The goal of the game is to "stay within the lines" defined by the high and low alert settings. Try this with your little gamer: turn the receiver on it's side and just observe the alert lines and the dots. Looks like a game to me. Some children might simply dismiss the idea, but others might be intrigued by it and (like me) they see this as a personal challenge. It's absolutely essential that the Surfer in training not be too harshly judged on his or her performance. Recognizing the effort is what's most important. This is one secret to achieving highly effective long term CGM use in children (and most other ages for that matter): the principle of NOT JUDGING.

Kevin McMahon conducted an interesting experiment with his teenage daughter with diabetes who had recently obtained a CGM device. His challenge was straightforward: to keep all her CGM readings between 60 mg/dL (3.3 mmol/L) and 200 mg/dL (11.1 mmol/L) for one 24 hour period. If she did that, he would reward her with $100 USD (roughly 68 GBP).

About one week later, she glowingly presented him with a 24 hour sensor track that met his challenge. Of course she got her reward, but Kevin's point was to help her learn a very valuable lesson. He asked her "What did you learn from this little challenge?". Her answer, insightful for a 15 year old teen, was "Well…I learned that I can do anything with my diabetes if I only put my mind to it".

Wisdom like this is achieved at different ages. Plus the ability to maintain an ongoing personal attention to self-care requires emotional maturity for sure. Effectively managing diabetes in children and teens is a team effort in every sense. Praise the child or teen for the effort, not the outcomes. Find the positives; don't dwell on the shortcomings or imperfections. These are the secrets to empowering children (and

adults) with any self-managed chronic illness.

Don't become the "sensor police"

Using a CGM in a child or teen as a "gotcha" tool is the best way to discourage its use. Watching large shifts (flux) in sugar levels occurring through the day may be disconcerting for some parents. Talk with your kid about what was going on but don't judge. Remember that while glycemic wave patterns may look similar from situation to situation, no two are ever exactly alike. But that's not important since Sugar Surfers are always on the move and can learn how to recover from an under or over treatment situation as long as they keep their eye on the trend line (see Pivoting).

A person with diabetes (of any age) cannot "will" their BG to be whatever they wish no matter how hard they try. Sugar levels are in constant motion in the human body. The creation of BG meters helped create a static mindset attitude towards BG levels. When asked, many younger children with diabetes believe that their blood sugar levels travel in straight lines like the charting software that comes from the meter companies. They might think the BG at 7:30 AM is still valid an hour later. Try asking a child with diabetes what their blood sugar level is two hours after the last check (assuming they have not eaten). Many children will say it is still the same as it was at the last check since no food was eaten. This is part of the concrete style of thinking that many young children fall prey to.

It's only through a series of choices, actions and reactions that the direction of the BG trend line is manipulated. The empowered person with diabetes makes their best assessment of the situation, acts on these, and then watches the results as they happen, even applying more food or insulin as the trend line moves forward in time. If something is under or overestimated and led to the trend line moving quickly up or down, this is simply a learning experience, not a condemnation of their abilities. It's vital that parents avoid applying judgmental terms or disapproving looks when discussing BG data from any source (meter or

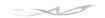

sensor). Take on the same mindset you did when teaching your child to ride a bicycle or throw a ball. You expected some falls and poor tosses, but that is the price of learning a useful new skill.

Tapping into hidden abilities

In my experience, most persons with diabetes possess the ability to sense changing blood sugar levels by subtle changes in their internal mental state of mind. I've learned there are areas of the brain that sense these changes in blood sugar levels. After decades of type 1 diabetes, I used to think that I had "hypoglycemia unawareness". For sure, the signs and symptoms that my body expresses a low BG has changed since I was young. Frankly, many of my natural internal alert mechanisms are not as strong as they used to be. But after I got my first real time CGM, I started to pay close attention to very subtle differences in the way my body felt when I knew my BG was dropping or rising quickly due to insulin, an activity, or after eating a large meal. As shifts in my BG were happening I glanced at the sensor readout pattern frequently.

As time went on and with lots of repetition, I became very proficient predicting whether my BG trend was rising, falling or simply tracking along a steady line. The process is easy. I stop, think "which direction is my BG moving?", then glance at the sensor readout to confirm my prediction. The sense of satisfaction I get when doing this makes me want to do it more as the day goes on. With practice and lots of repetition, I can now 'sense' a shifting BG trend when I am nowhere near the range of blood sugar considered hypoglycemic or hyperglycemic. For example, I'm able to sense a slight downward shift in BG from 130 mg/dL (7.2 mmol/L) to 120 mg/dL (6.7 mmol/L). It's not anything obvious to those watching me, like when I have a typical "mild" low BG event. It is my belief that almost all persons with diabetes possess this ability. But unlocking this remarkable ability requires a CGM device, lots of practice, time and attention. It's an amazing benefit of using a CGM that few discuss or even know about.

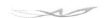

This page has been sponsored by: Dana Lynch

The sensor game

My little sensor game is something I do all the time. The object of the game is to mentally guess if my BG trend line is tracking steady, drifting down or rising quickly just before I glance at the sensor readout. As of this writing, I am 95% accurate in my predictions and some days close to 100% on the mark. But it took a while to develop this ability. It also took a lot of practice and patience. Today, I feel the cues of a drifting or dropping BG and verify the sensation by checking the sensor readout and checking a meter BG.

Try making up a "guess the trend" game of your own. It could just be something you do a few times each day with your child. The 3 answer options at first would be up, down or sideways (trending steady). Provide some form of low-cost reward for a correct answer, but don't react negatively in any way if the answer is incorrect. Every time the child correctly senses the trend line direction, they get a small reward of some type. The parent should randomly conduct the challenge through the day and check the sensor readout before quizzing the child about their sense of the situation. It's very important that this not be a game of "gotcha", so hold back on any verbal or non-verbal judgment of the readings. You are doing this only to exercise their ability to sense shifting blood sugar tides and to participate in their own care. Use only positive rewards and verbal reinforcement based on participation and not on blood sugar results.

The goal of the sensor game is to foster a sense of control and confidence in the child. After a while, these low cost rewards might get them practicing this skill on their own. Once they've developed competency in sensing a BG direction, you could take it to the next level by asking if they are drifting, dropping or spiking for extra bonus points. Hopefully, like me this becomes a personal challenge game that the child or teen does all the time whenever they prepare to check their sensor readout.

Learning from failure

A person with diabetes (of any age) cannot "will" their BG to be whatever they wish unless they fake the results. It's only through choices and actions that someone learns to control the direction of their BG trend line. The well supported child or teen with diabetes makes their best assessment of the situation, decides what to do, then acts on these decisions and watches the results as they occur. If they under or overestimated something that led to the trend line moving too quickly up or down, this is a learning experience, not a condemnation of their abilities. Failure is our best teacher. We just have to make sure our failed attempts are detected early and get promptly corrected. I can't overstate how very important it is for parents to absolutely avoid using judgmental words (or disapproving looks or glares) when dealing with BG data from a meter or a sensor. Put on your best poker face. Remember, there are no "good" or "bad" blood sugars. In range, high, low are fine terms to explain what is happening. Just don't judge.

Realistic expectations for raising Sugar Surfing kids

Sugar Surfing feeds on and generates self-confidence and creates a sense of empowerment. It takes time to achieve these feelings. Due to their youth and inexperience, children and teens might be more daring and willing to take greater risks. At first, they may lack a working understanding of the abstract properties and effects of insulin, food, exercise and stress on blood sugar. Parents must first possess this understanding before they can mentor their children. It's very misleading to equate diabetes independence with the ability to perform diabetes self-care actions such as injecting insulin or checking a blood sugar level. Parents should not just issue orders or reminders, but demonstrate and explain how the forces operate that move sugar levels in different directions. Sugar Surfing with kids is a team effort!

Expect the unexpected

Parents must also teach their children that unpredictable things can happen and not be surprised when unexpected BG drops or drifts

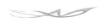

occur. Being better prepared for the unexpected reduces the chances of a bad outcome. Embracing the unpredictability of diabetes is hard to do at any age. As we learned in "False Idols", a + b does not always equal c. The ability to recognize and respond to unexpected drifting and shifting BG trends requires that parents and children develop an appreciation of the natural variability that is part of type 1 diabetes care. Empower your child by sharing the False Idols with them. They may say, "I told you so" and they would be right.

Setting high and low alert limits

Kids may need their low and high alert alarms set differently than grownups. For example, some children are very hard to treat when they are low; they fight and refuse to eat. In these cases, setting a higher "low" alert limit to reduce the chances of even a mild low would help until the child gets older and better able to deal with it, and the parents too! On the other hand, some children get very hyperactive and even unreasonable when their sugar is high, but are often much easier to treat when they get low. In these cases setting a lower "high" alert setting can reduce the number of harder to treat high BG spells. As kids get older these things may get better, but having the ability to adjust when the CGM alerts you about a high or low that may be coming can make a big difference in your life and the life of the child.

Aim at higher and wider BG target ranges when first starting to surf. For a small child, a lower limit for the alert threshold might be set at 100 mg/dL (5.6 mmol/L) and 250 mg/dL (13.9 mmol/L) for the high alert, possibly a bit higher. Aim to keep most readings in the mid to upper 100's (8 – 10 mmol/L). As greater proficiency is achieved, these margins can be made more narrow, but discuss with your doctor first. These BG margins are just guides. Just because you might go outside them occasionally is not a harmful thing so long as you steer them back into your zone using basic Sugar Surfing methods.

Don't make it too hard to win! Too narrow a BG target range results in frequent alarms, alarm fatigue, and eventually frustration. Aim to get

This page has been sponsored by: Christel Marchand Aprigliano

competent in keeping 75% or more of your tracings within a wide range at first. As confidence grows in your ability to do this, only then should you consider narrowing your margins.

Rate of change alarms can be set with different levels of sensitivity. In younger children, BG can drop really quickly as discussed above. Set the alert sensitivity to its highest level when first starting out. Also, glance at the CGM screen fairly often at first until you have a good understanding of your child's patterns of rise and fall in response to his/her various daily activities, meals and snacks. Like with anyone else, you might be more vigilant before, during, and after meal times. But afternoon play and sleep might reveal unexpected drops or rises too. Remember to confirm these data with your meter.

Change your targets to match the situation

Most great Sugar Surfing kids and families I know work to steer trending blood sugars towards an agreed upon desired BG target range. This target range can shift in size based on the situation (e.g., sleeping, on the playground, in school studying, competing at a sporting event, at a party). They use their sensor and meter to accomplish this, plus their experience and a commitment to follow through with ongoing checks after each action performed. It's also important to be able to watch a trend, determine its most likely cause, act to change it with exercise, food, insulin or a combination of each, and then follow through with more glances and corrective actions as needed downstream. Sugar Surfing is an action that continually repeats itself. Like exercising a muscle, daily Sugar Surfing skills gets stronger as you use them regularly.

Pivoting is more challenging

The action of making small, frequent diabetes self-management adjustments aimed at targeting a specific BG "bull's eye" is one way to describe the term pivoting. Adjustments used are numerous and described throughout this book. They are all based on careful watching (glancing) of the BG trend line on a well calibrated CGM device.

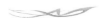

Tight pivoting requires experience with most of the Sugar Surfing methods you read about in Chapter 7 – How to Surf.

I consider this an advanced Sugar Surfing strategy that only a few highly motivated teens or closely monitored children might benefit from. Children and teens should usually aim to keep their BG levels in a zone or range rather than pivot around a specific target number.

The idea of a target is used with persons on the insulin pump or multi-dose insulin therapy (shots). It is an assigned value that is used to calculate a correction dose of rapid-acting insulin whenever a BG is out of range. Unfortunately, many patients are only taught to use this correction insulin calculation at meal time, in combination with the insulin taken for the carbs to be eaten. Correction insulin between meals might be forbidden by some physicians. Pivoting applies the concepts of well-practiced micro-dosing to steer out of range BG values discovered by frequent sensor glances back towards a central target value. This still results in the BG tracing existing within a "range" but the range is often much tighter when this method is done well.

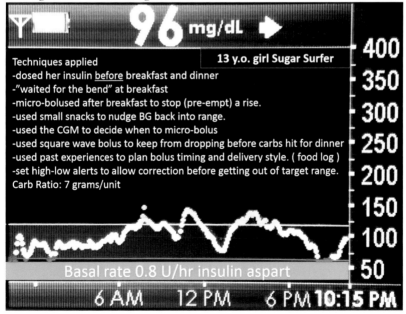

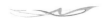

As you can tell, pivoting is a very high end Sugar Surfing strategy and only within the reach of the most highly motivated and well supported teen surfer. Here is an example of a 13 year old who is able to pull this off. I hope to see more teens Surfing like this as my method becomes embraced by more families.

Sensor fatigue

Brace yourself for sensor fatigue. You are seeing much more blood sugar data than ever before. Much of it will at first surprise you. Start to profile common daily situations and circumstances to characterize what happens to sugar levels in the blood. Share "sensor watch duty" with a spouse or other family member. One of the greatest drawbacks of sensors is also its strength: the constant flow of data. Loved ones need to develop the ability to know what is important to act on immediately and what can simply be watched. Nevertheless, in the current era of total data immersion this can bewilder many well intentioned parents and kids. The key is not to dwell but simply move on and re-glance later. Aim to be satisfied with BG tracks that stay in your zone most of the time. Straight line BG tracings are a bonus but not to be expected each day.

Kids and nighttime lows

For persons worried about low blood sugars being deadly, this is extremely rare. Internet posts can take a rare occurrence and blow it way out of proportion and frighten many people. The fact is that not every low is going to be deadly. There is a pervasive notion in some parent's mind that if you catch a 40 mg/dL (2.2 mmol/L) going down and treat it, that if you had not caught it the child would have died. Let me say that in my 30 plus years working with thousands of children with diabetes I've seen many hypoglycemic kids and adults below 40 mg/dL in many times. Many had no symptoms and easily recovered. Others passed out or had a seizure like episode and fully recovered. I've even been in this situation personally a number of times in the past as well. I can attest to the fear it creates, believe me.

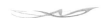

I'm not saying this to be cavalier about low blood sugars, but a reality check is needed here. The body has many internal defenses to protect the body from a low blood sugar. In fact these start happening as the blood sugar is dropping, starting in the 60-65 mg/dL range (3.3 - 3.5 mmol/L). But since it takes time for the body to rally, the person might still get a BG level low enough to cause them to pass out, collapse or have a low BG seizure. Sugar Surfing is one path to reducing the risk for severe lows in persons of all ages.

Timing is everything

Take the mealtime insulin dose before the meal when appropriate. Some families have fallen into a habit of dosing all insulin after the meal. This often allows the BG to rise higher than if the dose is taken prior to eating and you "wait for the bend". But children may not have the time or inclination to wait and will simply dose and eat... or eat then dose. Just keep this in mind when you review the after meal BG profile that follows. And remember why this is important: the lower the A1C level becomes, the more dependent it is on the quality of BG control AFTER the meal, not before.

When A1C values are 7.3% or lower, two-thirds of the value is the result of how well after meal BG levels are controlled, But when A1C is 10.3% or higher, this relations reverses; only one-third of the A1C results stems from the after meal BG levels with two-thirds coming from the pre-meal BG level of control.

If you micro-dose, check BG with a meter, watch the BG response to the small carb or small insulin dose, and verify the results in 2 - 3 hours with your meter. Many might avoid doing between meal corrections until other Surfing skills are mastered. Given how erratic most kids can be and how most will not be thinking about their BG control between meals, it's better to be conservative in this Surfing skill. You might choose to correct a sustained, straight trend line high BG with a standard correction dose as prescribed by your doctor or diabetes team. When you do this, up your game and "take the drop" carefully. Set

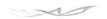

your lower BG alert limit a bit higher to give yourself a chance to prevent a low by treating with fast acting carbs before BG trends go too low. Check with your meter to verify.

Most successful families with Sugar Surfing kids typically act to steer trending blood sugars towards a desired target range. This range can shift based on the situation (e.g., sleeping, on the playground, in school studying, competing at a sporting event, at a party). They use their sensor, meter, experience and a commitment to follow through with ongoing checks after each action performed. It's also important to be able to watch a trend, determine its most likely cause and act with exercise, food, insulin or a combination of each. Follow through with more glances and corrective actions as needed.

"Aim small, miss small"

Micro-dosing small children with insulin or carbs might require fractions of units and only a few carbs to see significant shifts in the direction of the trend line. The idea of "aiming small" is a valuable concept in children. During basic diabetes education, we are taught to treat low blood sugar in children and adults the same way: with 15 grams of fast acting carbs. In the non-Sugar Surfing world, this boilerplate approach served a purpose. But in the CGM enabled world, many of you will find 15 grams to sometimes be far more than needed to raise a BG level from the hypoglycemic range. There will always be examples of when you might need that much and more to turn around a falling BG trend. The Rule of 15 is just another of many examples of static thinking that permeate diabetes care as discussed in chapter 5, False Idols.

Insulin sensitivity

Another challenge in younger children with diabetes is how sensitive their bodies can respond to insulin, especially when they are pre-school age. Insulin pumps have a feature called the duration of insulin action or active insulin time. In general, people who are resistant to the effect of insulin are assigned a short active insulin time

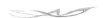

(2 - 3 hours). Persons who are sensitive to insulin are better suited for a longer time period. Parents who are setting the pump's insulin duration to 2 hours in little children raise the chances of giving more insulin than the child might need and increase the chances of low blood sugar. Most toddlers are better served by a longer active insulin time in their pump. If more insulin is needed for food or a high BG, it's better to make a choice to override the pump calculator and reduce the dose than to follow through on the pump calculator which might recommend giving more insulin than needed due to a short active insulin time programmed in the pump.

Many kids also don't wait to eat after they get an insulin dose. Many families see mid-morning blood sugar spikes that happen because of this. They usually come down. But some parents might choose to change the insulin to carbohydrate ratio instead of "waiting for the bend". The down side of this can be a risk of getting a low mid-morning blood sugar. One other reason for mid-morning spikes in some children has to do with the types of foods some of them like to eat, like processed breakfast cereals and milk.

Adhesives

More people are using glucose sensors than ever before. One significant problem is the growing number of kids and adults getting a skin rash or irritation to the tape adhesive that affixes the sensor apparatus on the skin. The medical term for this is contact dermatitis. It's also a problem that has plagued insulin pump users for years. In fact this is so common now that there are online support groups dedicated to sharing tips on how to best deal with the problem. In the worst case it might mean not being able to wear a sensor in one location for more than a few days at a time, which can run up the cost a lot. Most users try a variety of different adhesive tapes to wear as a barrier between the sensor adhesive and the skin. The use of steroid creams is problematic since prolonged use can be hurtful to the skin and in some cases get absorbed into the body and cause problems. I recently heard of successful use of intranasal steroid sprays (like fluticasone) as an

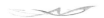

option to spray on the site before insertion (but clean the site thoroughly before placing the sensor). I suggest finding a good medical supply store (even online) and investigate tape options for persons with tape sensitivity problems. Cut pieces into small strips and apply them into an area you don't use for the sensor and see if a skin reaction occurs over time. Some areas of the body might be less prone to react due to skin thickness. Therefore moving the site to the hip or thigh might work as opposed to the abdomen or arm. But if all these efforts fail you might be unable to wear a sensor until the companies come up with less allergenic adhesives.

What if my child doesn't want to Surf yet?

If you have a child with diabetes at any age who is unwilling (or unable) to tolerate wearing a sensor, you might just have to check BG levels very often to get the necessary information, perhaps as often as 12 - 16 times daily. In these situations some Sugar Surfing basics can still be applied, such as tracking basal insulin steadiness by frequent review of collected BG data charts each day, dosing insulin in front of a meal (based on the pre-meal BG level), checking BG levels 2-3 hours after the meal, and even applying small doses of corrective insulin or micro-carbing to prevent lows between meals. But you must be able to check BG frequently enough after any corrective insulin or carbohydrate dosing to see if the desired BG outcome was achieved a few hours later. This helps to prevent an over or under-correction. It all comes down to how much information you can gather and how well you can apply it "in the moment" to steer the blood sugar data trend. This amount of mental involvement and frequent BG checking is hard for many young people to sustain. But even if you only focus on before and after meal BG control and improved insulin timing before a meal, you will see a benefit in overall glucose control. So you don't absolutely need a CGM device to Sugar Surf, but it does make many management decisions much easier to make.

If your child with diabetes has zero interest in a sensor or Sugar Surfing, don't despair. Their attitudes may change with time. Don't try

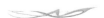

and force the issue. It may only backfire. Sugar Surfing is intended to empower people. It's hard to feel empowered when something has been forced onto you. Of course younger kids might just go along for the ride and grow into appreciating their CGM's but that is not guaranteed.

The principles of care that form the basis of this discipline also cross over to improve conventional management. My co-author and I proved this in a randomized clinical trial we published in 2012. This formed the basis of "Frequent Pattern Management" which was the philosophical forerunner of Sugar Surfing. What we found in that study was that families who reviewed meter based blood sugar patterns at least once per week had lower A1C results compared to those who reviewed their own data less than once per week. What was also enlightening was that those families who did perform reviews every few weeks were no better off than those who performed no review at all. Being thoughtful about your blood sugars at least once per week seems to be one key to better blood sugar control. The BG data you collect must be put back into making better self-care choices 'in the moment' or if using a meter, review at least once a week and repeat the cycle.

Surfing through the kitchen and the pantry

I've written a book that has not given much attention to a major element of how diabetes is controlled: by careful attention to what and how much is eaten each day. That is my bad, especially since one of my children is a Registered Dietitian. That said, this book is nearly 300 pages already so let's focus on that for perhaps the next book in a series. Let me say here that every family with a child with diabetes should have access to a diabetes educator and a registered dietitian. Ongoing diabetes education is the best defense against this disease.

Most children and teens have food preferences that repeat themselves. For example, some kids eat the same 5 things for breakfast and the same 6 things for lunch and so on. This predictability can be turned into a great advantage. It allows for the ability to "learn" the

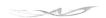

typical blood sugar response to that meal (or snack). I advise my families to use the "top ten" principle to hone in on the most commonly eaten meals and snacks that are prepared during the week. The CGM results from each insulin and meal "attempt" is then used to create a profile. Over time and with practice you create a personal library of actions or steps which involve not only how much insulin is needed, but how it is best delivered (standard injection, combination or extended bolus [pump] or using an "I-chain" (see Appendix).

I'm not dismissing carb counting and I'm not advocating any particular meal plan or diet. In fact, carb counting is very important but it's just a starting point. Sugar Surfing takes this further. If the BG profile that follows a carefully calculated and timed insulin dose and meal is observed, and the after meal BG pattern was what you desired, then this same approach should be used the next time this same meal is eaten. If there was a high or low after the meal, then an adjustment should be made on the next try. This approach works best when the food is measured or comes from a package with standard servings. You might also say "change the carb ratio" and you might get the result you want with this particular meal. But that might not work with another type or amount of food. Carb ratios are discussed in Chapter 5.

It is well known that many children poorly measure food or count carbs well. In these situations, it may require 'in the moment' decisions based on rapidly rising BG levels after the meal. Dosing additional insulin in these cases is an advanced step and I discuss this in detail in Chapter 14.

If you choose not to prevent a spike in progress, be sure to make changes next time when you attempt this same meal. The images on the next page   shows my strategy for determining the optimal insulin dosing strategy for a popular children's cereal.

In this example, the results of the first attempt were used to change the second attempt the next day.

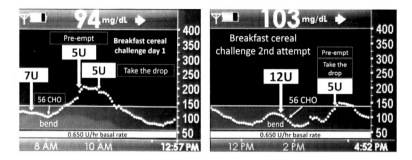

By the third attempt I had crafted an effective approach to this food. This same principle is used for any new food or meal. It just takes the three virtues to pull it off.

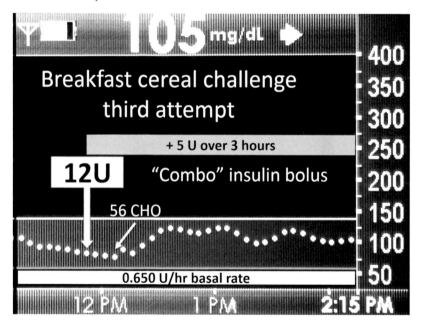

Sugar Surfing allows us to better choreograph or balance the effects of food and insulin on blood sugar trends. Insulin dosing formulas are modified as needed based on close observation of the BG trend line. The experience gained from each attempt with the child or teen is immediately fed forward to improve the results of the next attempt. It's a cycle of continuous improvement.

Sugar Surfing in children versus the world of diabetes medicine

This true story was shared with me by a mom who has closely followed and used Sugar Surfing techniques with her teen daughter.

"Hi Dr. Ponder! I want to share an interesting story with you. Yesterday was our pediatric endocrinologist visit. By the way, it always causes severe anxiety for me (and always has despite repeatedly good A1C's). It's as if I have PTSD from my Abigail's diagnosis 5 years ago. Anyhow, our CDE/RN walked in the room and said to my Abigail, 'Everything looks great with your control but I see a few strange things that I have never seen in a pumper in all my years of looking at downloads. By the way, who mostly manages your diabetes Abigail?' Abigail responded, 'Me.' The CDE said, 'I see a ton on activity on here indicating temporary basal rates and mini bolusing. You need to be a kid. Don't you feel tethered to your pump? You shouldn't be making those changes. Temp basals are for exercise only.' Abigail said, 'Well, no, I just make a decision and move on.' Now, in full disclosure, I surfed for her until I felt comfortable turning it over to her.

Unfortunately, lately, she has over corrected several times. We are backing off a bit to revisit our correction factors. But she rocked a 6.3 (mmol/l [113 mg/dL]. I was shocked. Proud and shocked. I am leery of pushing below 6 at this time but I truly am ultra-happy at 6.3. All smiles. True story. Have a great day."

Most people who Sugar Surf are going to challenge the training and experience of many excellent diabetes care providers. Sugar Surfing is the ultimate expression of individualized care fueled by empowerment and teamwork within a family as illustrated above. This is why I find this anecdote a bit ironic, given that all major diabetes organizations advocate individualized care for every patient. But be prepared for push back by well-intentioned health care providers. This book is intended to raise everyone's awareness, not serve as a prescribed course of action. Use what you learn here to start a discussion with your diabetes team. In time, I believe Sugar Surfing will become embraced

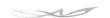

by the medical establishment. This book and my workshops are how I plan to get this modern approach to the masses.

Attitude rules!

A parent best promotes CGM acceptance in their child by using the data from these devices in a non-judgmental fashion. One goal of Sugar Surfing should be early detection and recognition of significant BG trending patterns as they occur. This allows the child and parent to make prudent self-care decisions to blunt or re-direct the trend line away from low or high BG target ranges as they happen in real time. This requires good open communication between parent and child. If the parent shows disdain or disapproval of a rapidly rising or falling BG, even a comment like "What's this?" could be interpreted negatively by the child, who might be less inclined to share next time. Approach the CGM data your child shares with you with a sense of exploration and as a partner, not a judge. Some parents may struggle with this approach more than the child. Many successful Surfing families will attest that this is the secret to high quality family-centered Sugar Surfing.

We all fall off the path of tight blood sugar control, all of us, from time to time. That doesn't make us bad, it just makes us human. I'm no different. There are days where I'm a lot more careful and picky than others with my BG control. And there are some days when I'm very careful and selective about what and how much I eat. But I also have days when I want to eat anything and everything I want, lay around and do nothing, and skip meals. But I still try to keep a close eye on my sensor readout and use what I've learned to keep my BG tracings in range. But I still have roller coaster days like everyone else and you will too.

I think the basic principles of Sugar Surfing are ideal for children. Surfing builds a foundation for achieving tighter BG control that can grow with the child, plus it encourages the family to remain active in their care. Contrast this to the days when only BG meter checks were

used and the information gathered was largely ignored or reviewed months later when it would have no impact.

I'm confident that if you incorporate these suggestions into your thinking and consistently use them with your child or teen with diabetes, you can break through those barriers which may be holding you back now. Team surfing with your child takes patience and a tolerance. Mistakes will be made and much can be learned from them. Just remember not to judge yourself too harshly (or your youngster). Learn from the failed effort how to best prepare for the next attempt and always keep trying.

Staying engaged

Sugar Surfing is all about learning how to use a set of tools to influence the direction of a person's blood sugar trend. It only takes 5 seconds and I can be doing other things while I'm doing it. It's just part of being aware of the situation. If I see something on the trend line that concerns me, I'll stop what I'm doing and give it more thought.

Remote monitoring and surfing: "Calling it in?"

There are now devices which permit remote observers to check another person's BG meter results or CGM device readouts in real time. Most of these devices reside in the hands of parents or adult children of older persons with diabetes. Mainly the former. So we are already in the era of continuous BG data streaming to others, usually family members. This is yet another way Sugar Surfing can occur as a team activity between the patient and the patient's personal care team (usually their family) and at any age enabled by easy access to wireless devices to make communicating between family members easier.

The key to real-time remote diabetes care is accurate and timely two-way communication. Watching a CGM from a distance is one thing. Inserting yourself into the moment from far away is something entirely different and demands that you have more information than just a blood sugar reading. In this era of virtual care, make sure you don't

make too many assumptions and ensure that the BG situation is fully understood before making decisions which could impact your child. For example, all of us have experienced the limitations inherent in text messaging as a form of communication. When it's time for a conversation don't hesitate to make the call. As Sugar Surfers know, it's not just about what goes into an action but just as important is assessing the result of those actions. In other words, don't assume that what you agreed to do in advance with your remote child or teen with diabetes actually occurred.

Children can sugar surf at any age. Active family involvement and non-judgmental emotional support are necessary for long term success. Finding ways to encourage the child to wear the sensor and effectively use the data it provides are the greatest start up challenges for the family. As with any practicable skill, it takes patience, consistency and resilience to become a good Sugar Surfing family. Diabetes care is the sum of your choices; the ones you act on as well as the ones you don't. You don't send a child to surf in the ocean without an instructor, lifeguard or experienced surf buddy always present. Children best surf with decision support and encouragement from those who know them best: their families.

This page has been sponsored by: Austin Enerson

Sharks in the Water

Chapter 9

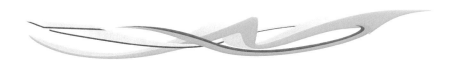

Now that you know the why and the how of Sugar Surfing let's focus a bit on trouble shooting a situation you likely know something about but may not have an in-depth understanding: KETONES.

You may have encountered them a few times in the past. These are what I call "sharks in the water". Like sharks in the ocean, ketones are always around and usually leave us alone. Ketones are actually part of our normal metabolism and we depend on them much more than you realize, especially overnight. For these reasons, all Sugar Surfers need a good working understanding about ketones.

Just in case you're a bit rusty or didn't know this, ketones are always inside us. It's only a matter of how much. Ketones are small molecules that serve as a low energy cellular energy source. The brain and other tissues can use ketones as an energy source instead of sugar. During long periods of fasting (not eating), our bodies use ketones to conserve blood sugar. They will increase in quantity under certain circumstances in both diabetic and non-diabetic individuals. Unfortunately, we are often taught to fear all ketones.

This is unfortunate since these are otherwise harmless chemicals under most circumstances. There are several ketone forms in our blood: beta hydroxybutyrate, acetoacetic acid and acetone. We should respect, not fear, ketones. Just to illustrate that ketones and normal blood sugar peacefully coexist, here is a side by side image of my morning BG on the right and ketone level using a blood ketone 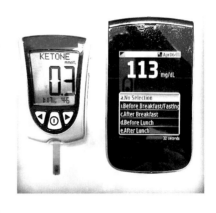 meter. As you can see here, some ketones are always present.

The following scenario is an example of a normal ketone situation. I was called about a teen with type 1 diabetes who was discovered to have large ketones in urine and a BG (rechecked) in the 150 mg/dL (8.3 mmol/L) range. This teen was not in diabetic ketoacidosis (DKA), but had not eaten much food over the last couple of weeks due to a surgical procedure. In order to meet his body's energy needs, his system converted other substances in the body (mainly body fat) into a source of usable cellular energy, better known as ketones. The fact that his blood sugar was in a reasonable range (under 200 mg/dL [11.1 mmol/L]) shows that his cells can take up sugar (glucose) for energy because there was sufficient insulin in the teen's system to allow this to happen. In this case the presence of ketones was a normal adaptation to under-eating (mostly lack of carbohydrates). Note the absence of high blood sugar and dehydration. This boy was not in DKA.

High blood or urine ketones don't always equal diabetic keto-acidosis, but they always require close attention. In this case the family contacted the diabetes doctor by phone just to be safe. They verified the

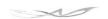

teen was not nauseated or vomiting. That meant it was safe to continue his management at home. In this case, additional water intake and monitoring was recommended to help flush the ketones out of the system through the urine. Had the teen been nauseated, more aggressive steps would have been needed (such as anti-nausea therapy, staying well hydrated with water or other liquids, frequent BG checking and extra rapid-acting insulin doses as needed) to keep BG levels in a reasonable range (under 200 mg/dL [11.1 mmol/L]).

The most common mistakes made by persons with type 1 diabetes faced with mild illness situations like this are:

1. Not checking BG often enough after a high BG is first discovered;

2. Not checking ketones after starting treatment until they're unmeasurable;

3. Not giving extra rapid-acting insulin as instructed by the diabetes team;

4. Not drinking adequate fluids to stay properly hydrated;

5. Not treating nausea early; and,

6. Waiting too long to call the care team for advice.

Diabetic ketoacidosis (DKA)

When insulin levels in the blood of a person with type 1 diabetes fall too low, the breakdown of fat into ketones goes up dramatically, literally flooding the body with more ketones and their byproducts than can be safely used as an energy source. The low amount of effective insulin on board makes the blood sugar rise. Without enough insulin to move sugar into cells, glucose travels 'round and 'round the blood stream until it finds an exit in the urine. The high sugar levels force the body to use water to remove the excess sugar. In doing so, the person is at risk for dehydration unless enough water can be consumed to prevent it. The high sugar level and the increased output of urine also

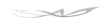

makes the person thirsty. This high sugar, high urine output, high water intake situation may continue for a long time. But without enough insulin to shut off excess ketone production, matters worsen and chemical byproducts of out of control ketone formation act on the intestines and the brain to induce nausea. The nauseated person slows down drinking, yet the loss of water does not slow down. The end result is more water leaving the body than coming into it. Dehydration is not far behind. And dehydration itself acts as a stress on the body that generates more ketones. At this point the process feeds back on itself in a downward spiral making diabetic ketoacidosis imminent. The only way to stop it from happening is to take insulin as often as needed and stay well hydrated. Managing nausea early on can also buy time for extra insulin doses to stop ketones from being formed and lower the blood sugar levels slowing down this vicious cycle. Sadly, many persons don't recognize this problem is upon them until it's too late. In those cases, the only remaining option is a trip to the hospital or emergency department.

Ketones are misunderstood

Ketones are often referred to in a negative light by persons with type 1 diabetes. All you low-carb dieters out there are well-versed on what ketones are and their relevance. Low carbohydrate diets are designed to promote the formation of ketones in blood. Without dietary carbohydrates to trigger an insulin response, the body is able to break down fat for energy. This is because high insulin levels block fat breakdown. Anything that lowers insulin levels in the blood, or drives up stress hormones, tends to trigger the breakdown of fat for energy. Ketones are the result of that process. The presence of ketones is an indicator that fat is being consumed.

In fact, since urine strips report the term "negative", this further fuels the misconception. I advise against believing a person "never" gets ketones. Ketones are not checked with the same frequency as blood sugar levels and many who feel they don't even generate them might be surprised if they only had more information. I think we all know that

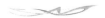

statements which include "never" and "always" can be too broad. And it's more than dislodged insulin pump sites that cause a ketone/high BG situation with a pump. Don't forget air gaps in pump tubing and insulin leaking back around the catheter (tunneling), too! The most common reason is skipping scheduled insulin doses either by accident or intentionally.

Prudence and situational thinking are necessary to understand ketones and their significance. Remember, almost everyone wakes up with a tiny amount of ketones in the blood from not eating for several hours. Their presence is simply part of the body adapting to a mild fast, even in persons with type 1 diabetes.

I recommend you become a student (of sorts) regarding ketones. Learn when they are relevant to the situation and when they are not. Most of all, don't panic. Learn the "sick day" care rules and refer to them whenever you feel the need. You don't need to be "sick" to make use of these rules. The purpose of these guidelines is to prevent high BG and ketones from turning into a feeding frenzy on your well controlled diabetes. The better you understand your foe, the less scary it starts to seem.

Ketones get all the blame

Patients with diabetes are taught to check for urine or blood ketones when illness strikes or when the BG is high (usually 250 mg/dL [13.9 mmol/L] or higher). If ketones are elevated this is taught as a "bad thing". I won't debate that here, but ketones take the blame for too much that goes wrong in diabetic ketoacidosis. Let me explain why.

Ketones are the byproducts of rapid breakdown of body fat due to a relative (or absolute) lack of insulin. But ketones are not the only byproduct of this process. Other biologically active compounds, known broadly as prostaglandins [specifically, prostacyclin (PGI2) and dinoprostone (PGE2)], are greatly overproduced by fat cells when there is not enough insulin on board. This happens within 3 hours of withdrawal of insulin from a person with type 1 diabetes. These

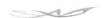

chemicals cause diabetic blood vessels to dilate (open up) during DKA, which is why persons in DKA typically appear flushed and warm to the touch, as opposed to cold and clammy due to other types of body dehydration.

When extra insulin is given by injection, the levels of these blood vessel dilating prostaglandins starts to drop. Prostaglandins are also largely responsible for the nausea, vomiting, and stomach pain that occur with ketosis. Anything that prevents a person from taking in fluids can worsen their dehydration.

So don't blame the lowly ketone for nausea and vomiting. In some ways it's an innocent bystander. The ketones themselves aren't making you feel as nauseated as you think, it's the prostaglandins. Since we can't measure prostaglandins with a meter or urine test, ketones will continue to take the heat for all the things that go wrong in DKA. However, high ketones do contribute to the acid level buildup in blood and stir up other metabolic problems, but NOT all the nausea and vomiting.

Under normal conditions the body requires about one tenth (10%) of the amount of "effective" insulin action to prevent uncontrolled ketone production and, ultimately, diabetic ketoacidosis (DKA) compared to the amount of insulin to manage a rising level of sugar coming into the bloodstream from a meal. Anti-insulin hormones such a glucagon, play a role in driving DKA too, not just a lack of insulin action or effect. Studies done long ago showed that if glucagon was chemically blocked from being released and insulin was kept very low, DKA took days to occur as opposed to hours. This means that the presence of ketones (high amounts, not small amounts) in blood or urine suggests a state of high insulin need.

The sharks of hubris

The word hubris means excessive pride or self-confidence. This word applies to how some persons approach ketone management or other aspects of their own self-care. Hubris is a very powerful shark in

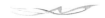

the water. Here are some statements of hubris I have heard over the years from persons with type 1 diabetes. Have you ever heard (or said) something similar?

"She never has ketones when she's sick."

"I've never been in DKA. I think I'm resistant to it."

"The glucagon is expired but she's never had severe low blood sugar anyway."

"I know the exact carbs in that number one burger meal, I found it on the internet."

"I've got two dollars with me in case I get low during my run."

"The meter says 384 (21.3 mmol/L), but why is he twitching and acting low?"

"I just miss a few shots a week, what difference does that make?"

"Exercise always lowers my blood sugar."

"It's ok to take my insulin now, this restaurant always serves their meals fast."

"I'm ok, leave me alone."

"I'm not low...my hair always stands on end like this."

I've had type 1 diabetes for decades. The only time I went into DKA was when I ran out of insulin in college and made the mistake of thinking I could go a day without it. That was a huge mistake. I spent three days in the hospital. But I learned a valuable lesson that I never repeated and I learned how to keep the DKA sharks at bay. In my defense I had never been taught what would happen if I didn't take my insulin. Diabetes education was a largely self-taught process in the 1960's and 70's where I lived. But I fell prey to a false assumption.

Unfortunately we often place TOO much trust in our personal assumptions. It's in those over confident moments that we become most vulnerable to the sharks in the water.

Good Sugar Surfers always play it safe. But many surfers want to push the envelope and take their skills to the next level. That requires a willingness to push the limits and try new things. In a later chapter I will discuss how to safely experiment with diabetes control with the least risk possible. But if you're not inclined to try freestyling it, basic Sugar Surfing can still be of great help.

Riptides & Sandbars

Chapter 10

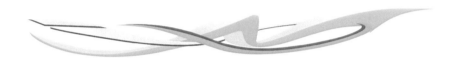

Now that you know the why and the how of Sugar Surfing, let's focus a bit on trouble-shooting several situations that may undermine your Sugar Surfing and cause you to fall off your board temporarily or wipeout altogether. You may have encountered them in the past. Many are common problems, actions, or inactions encountered by persons with diabetes taking insulin. All are manageable and most are preventable. I call these situations "Riptides and Sandbars". Sugar Surfing will teach you how to recognize and avoid some of these hazards, and to get back on your surfboard if you fall off!

Omitting insulin doses

This is like diving off your board in the middle of a ride. At some point, persons with type 1 diabetes will eventually be late to take a scheduled insulin dose or simply forget to take a shot. I've missed shots before. And when I did it had consequences. The first time was when I was in college. I ran out of insulin over the weekend. Since I didn't fully understand what would happen if I missed a scheduled insulin dose, I just decided to wait until Monday to get a new vial of insulin. In the 1970's most pharmacies were closed on Sundays. As I shared in the previous chapter, I thought (very incorrectly) that I could miss my Sunday shot and simply restart it on Monday. I spent the next 3 days recovering from diabetic ketoacidosis (DKA) in the University infirmary. It was my first, and last, episode of DKA due to intentionally omitted insulin.

Omitted insulin is common, whether it's a shot or through a pump. This is the Sugar Surfer's strongest riptide. Sometimes the insulin is skipped on purpose. Taking little to no insulin for a low-carb meal is an example. In this case this choice is reasonable and will not cause problems. This only applies to meal time insulin. You would never want to stop a scheduled dose of long acting (basal) insulin.

Insulin omission is misused as a method to lose weight. It's a very dangerous thing to do and can result in serious long term consequences in regards to higher rates of diabetes complications and more frequent episodes of DKA. Skipping scheduled mealtime insulin doses devastates your immediate BG control. A more passive form of omission is when a high BG is measured and a choice is made NOT to take an insulin dose to correct that out of range BG value. Skipping insulin is the antithesis of Sugar Surfing.

Using old / outdated / heat damaged insulin

This undercurrent is more insidious that outright skipping a dose of inulin. It has many of the same results, but there is no obvious intent. You are often taking your insulin as suggested. But in this case, the insulin has been compromised by being outdated or somehow damaged by poor handling.

The best practice is to discard any open insulin vials after being used for 1 month. One tip is to write the opening date on the vial. After 4 weeks, make a point to discard that vial. This reduces the chances of

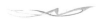

using insulin with less potent effect. If you look at your insulin and it appears discolored in any way or has matter floating in the vial, then consider discarding that insulin and opening a new vial.

This is an tricky problem because the loss of insulin strength is small at first. The higher BG levels that follow its use may be incorrectly believed to be due to other factors like overeating or stress.

Making an error in your insulin dose

This is an honest mistake for adults and most children and teens. Although there are formulas and charts to tell the patient how much insulin to self-administer, we can make an honest mistake and under-dose or even forget and over dose insulin. In families, one parent might give a scheduled dose, not tell the other parent, who then gives the same dose twice. The reverse can occur when one parent "thinks" the other dosed the child but in reality neither did and a high BG follows. Children or teens who are mostly in charge of their own insulin shots or pump boluses are notorious for making dosing errors.

The best solution is sharing dosing responsibilities and open communication about when shots are given. Insulin pumps have memories and the user can quickly check when the last dose was taken and how much. Many insulin pump users rarely check their pump histories, nor do their parents.

Improper pump programming / incorrect time on pump

In my practice, I sometimes find settings on insulin pumps that are improperly programmed. For some reason the basal rate is more than what it should be (or less). This could be the result of an error made when changing a setting. In other cases a child might have accidentally changed the settings. Keeping a written copy of the settings on a pump are very important but infrequently done.

A pump relies on a properly set internal clock time. All programmed changes in settings are cued to the pump clock. If using only a single basal rate, carb ratio and correction factor like me, the time on the

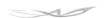

pump is not all that important. I once got a call from a noted pediatric endocrinologist regarding one of his patients using a pump. The boy was having frequent lows at night and highs during the day. As we went through all the possible explanations I could imagine, when I got down my list to checking the clock time, there was a long pause. "That's it", he said. The AM and PM had been switched and the higher daytime basal rate settings were happening at night, causing the frequent low BG's and wreaking havoc on his control and stressing him and his parents. About twice a year I still see complete AM and PM reversals on an insulin pump clock.

A more subtle problem arises when daylight savings time comes around. I often find patients who might go for weeks with the time set incorrectly on their pump after the time change. Again if there is only one basal rate this would really be of no consequence, but for others it could be significant if a scheduled basal rate change happens too early or later than it should.

Air bubbles (in "tubed" pumps) or kinked tubing

When loading a pump reservoir and priming the pump tubing, if proper care isn't used the system can be compromised. Air bubbles or air gaps in the tubing will result in lack of insulin of different spans of time based on the size of the air bubble or gap. This speaks to the need to take your time when replacing an insulin pump infusion site and loading a new reservoir and infusion set. Purge all the air from the tubing and out of the reservoir. Likewise, a kink in the tubing will prevent the insulin you program the pump to deliver from actually being infused, resulting in a lack of insulin and an unexpectedly elevated BG.

Malfunctioning pump site

Don't get distracted and forget an important step in the process, like this man did when he forgot to remove the cover cap on the pump catheter before inserting the set. The site never entered the skin. Within a couple of hours after attempting insertion, his BG skyrocketed. Notice

what his CGM registered afterwards and how he quickly recovered with injected insulin.

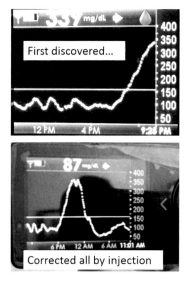

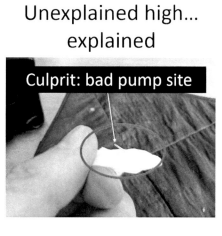

The best practice is to always check a BG level 2 hours after a site change. This provides a safety check that pump insulin is controlling BG levels, reassuring you that insulin is being infused properly under the skin by the catheter.

Tunneling

Tunneling is a phenomenon where insulin leaks back along the sides of an insulin catheter and onto the surface of the skin. This can happen in a catheter that has been in place for several days.

The skin around the catheter might have stiffened and lost the proper seal around the catheter. Insulin takes the path of least resistance.

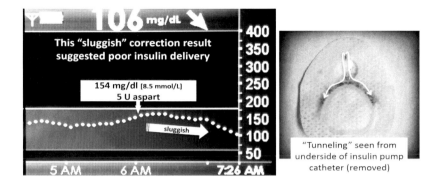

This "sluggish" correction result suggested poor insulin delivery

154 mg/dl [8.5 mmol/L]
5 U aspart

sluggish

"Tunneling" seen from underside of insulin pump catheter (removed)

The consequences are broad and potentially severe. Anywhere from mildly higher BG readings than normal to full blown high BG and ketones leading to DKA if not discovered soon enough.

Not changing insulin pump infusion site often enough/site infection

Insulin pump supplies are expensive. Sometimes persons will leave the infusion site in too long. This will cause redness and itching, which could be the first signs of a skin infection. As a site is starting to lose its integrity, the BG levels may start to trend higher. This might at first be blamed on other forces. But after inserting a fresh infusion site, the BG patterns might quickly drop into a more desirable range.

An infusion site infection is often the result of leaving a catheter in place too long. Poor site preparation or lack of sterile technique at insertion time can cause infections that could result in an abscess. Most pump site abscesses are due to Staph bacteria on skin. The pus should be properly drained by the health care provider and an antibiotic prescribed that covers most common skin bacteria. A culture of the pus will reveal if the bacteria is sensitive to the prescribed antibiotic. If not, the medication needs to be changed.

Not attempting to estimate carbs at meal/snack time

This is by far the greatest challenge for most persons with type 1 diabetes. Insulin is best balanced to the effect of the meal eaten. Insulin doses might be based on how much carbohydrate is within the meal to

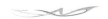

be eaten. If the carb count is wrong, or not even done, then it will be just blind luck if the BG levels that follow will be in any way "controlled".

Studies that investigated the carb counting abilities of adolescents showed a poor retention of these skills even after thorough training was offered and the teens were shown to be competent carb counters. After one month, less than one fourth of these teens could accurately count carbs in their favorite foods within 10 grams of the actual amount upon which they were tested.

Not "Waiting for the Bend"

In Chapter 7, How to Surf, you learned the value of timing insulin relative to food and how to "Wait for the Bend". Sometimes we're not able to wait and an insulin-food mismatch happens, which drives up the after meal BG higher than necessary. Not paying enough attention to matching insulin action to meals or snacks using your sensor as a guide invites excessive BG flux to occur. Since A1C values are heavily influenced by the after meal BG rise, a valuable method to rein in BG levels is missed.

Not glancing at the sensor readout often enough

The frequency that the BG readout is seen is the primary way the Sugar Surfer maintains situational awareness of their BG trends. If the readout is viewed infrequently or rarely, this acts to reduce the number of opportunities to steer the BG trend line. Many golden opportunities are missed. I teach Surfers to consider each glance at the CGM screen as pearl of great value. But that value is fleeting and must be spent in the moment. This book teaches how to use those data as effectively as possible, squeezing every bit of value from a BG reading and trend pattern. But not every glance requires action. Most of the time these are just "updates" for me. If I see the early stages of an emerging trend, I may glance more often. I don't want to get caught off guard. As more people use CGM devices with a phone or possibly a data-enabled watch, this skill will be easier to perform and practice.

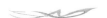

Ignoring BG trends on the sensor readout until too late

Ignoring BG trends and alert alarms is "playing chicken" with your control. Sugar Surfing is all about balancing the proactive and reactive elements of your self-management. Waiting too long to pre-empt (treat) a dropping BG trend puts you at risk for a severe low. Conversely, watching a double arrow rise in BG well past your highest alert threshold might put you in jeopardy for DKA from a bad pump site.

Ignoring high or low alerts

High and low alerts are set by you the CGM user. They can also be changed to meet the circumstances then changed back as needed. I don't mind using different high and low alerts for sleeping than I do for outdoor activity. When they go off, heed the alerts by checking your BG and doing an internal "gut check" to ask yourself if you can also sense the dropping or rising BG. Most of all, don't delay correcting the situation quickly and not postponing action. You do so at your own peril.

Poor calibration technique with your CGM

This is simple garbage in garbage out (GI-GO) thinking. Chapter 6, Waxing you Board, is dedicated to why proper calibration is so important to Sugar Surfing. Treat your CGM well and it will treat you well. Poor to non-existent CGM calibration undermines all you set out to do as a Surfer. Sloppy calibration methods are no further away than the next BG check.

Not calibrating your BG meter (per manufacturer's instructions)

Very few persons actually go to the trouble of calibrating their BG meter using proper control solution. Since these devices provide the data to be entered into a CGM device, another GI-GO cycle gets started here. As discussed in Chapter 5, False Idols, all BG meters have some error built into them. The only way variability is kept to a minimum is by practicing careful hand washing, proper sample collection, good strip handling and periodic meter calibration with control solution.

This page has been sponsored by: William C. Alger

Always believing your child or teen

At the risk of sounding indelicate, we all lie at some time in our lives. In fact most of us tell some sort of mistruth each day, sometimes many. Whole personas are built upon lies are spread across our history and in our fiction. In my diabetes practice I routinely come across children (and parents) with diabetes who misrepresent the truth to me in an interview. They lie. I can't always tell why, but I suspect it's often out of concern or fear of how I might react or judge them, make a condescending comment, or roll my eyes with frustration. And I will not lie here and tell you I've never done those things before. I've even lied to my own doctor in the past. We are all imperfect.

At diabetes camp, where I have served annually since 1981, I oversee the care of hundreds of children with diabetes from other parts of my state. The residential camp environment is unique. At camp, there is a greater feeling of acceptance and sense of belonging amongst the hundreds of boys and girls who attend annually. It's here that many of these children have shared their personal stories of lying to their parents and doctors to keep from being judged harshly, fabricated blood sugar data, or manipulated their diabetes to seek attention from others. One girl once told me the story about how she was punished and yelled at for any high blood sugars. Her response? Make up new ones.

Older children with diabetes usually know what worries and upsets their parents. While many will not go as far as to fabricate BG results, many choose to simply tell their loved one what they think they want to hear. If the parents are busy with their own lives, everyone stays happy and harmony is maintained. This harmony might be shattered at the next doctor visit when BG control is measured and does not match up with what is in writing, or what the child or teen verbally reports. If the A1C is in range, there is little reason for the doctor to question anyone's honesty even though lies and omissions may already be well established. These behaviors go undiscovered because they have not risen to a level that compromises the child's diabetes control.

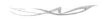

Many parents refuse to accept that their well-adjusted child with diabetes would lie to them and staunchly defend them to others when their child's actions are questioned. This is what parents should usually do, but they should also be mindful that the child or teen with diabetes might be putting up a stoic front because they might be over their head with daily self-care choices and not really know what to do. Asking the parent for help might only elicit a dismissing comment like "You should know how to do this by now", or "You need to grow up". Often lurking behind the confident veneer of a teen with diabetes might be a bundle of internal conflicts, including lingering fears and ongoing misunderstandings about diabetes. Some kids just choose to put only minimal effort into their diabetes as they struggle to grow up in an ever more complex world.

What living with diabetes fifty years has taught me is not to judge others struggling with my condition too harshly, or preferably not at all. This is why I tell all my children with diabetes and their families I will not judge them. I feel in approaching them this way I might reduce the number of mistruths, incomplete answers, and flat out lies that they might tell another doctor. In general this has been a great way to do business and has opened more doors into my patient's lives than it has closed. I do understand the challenge of living with diabetes each day and the hopes and fears that travel with me with every waking moment. I can relate, but I also want to keep it "real".

Parents should not expect kids to take on full control of their diabetes until at least age 16. Even this is an average. Some might be able to do it at younger ages. Many others need more time. Approach diabetes as a team effort from the beginning, share information openly and hold your tongue when you hear a child tell you they forgot to take a shot or bolus, or told you their BG was something it wasn't or simply made something up. It might be a sign you need to back up a bit and re-engage with you child or teen and share these diabetes duties. But again, don't judge harshly. Avoid the use of "good" and "bad" in reference to a number. Moralistic terms have no place in a diabetes discussion.

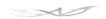

This page has been sponsored by: TJ Phillips

To be a good Sugar Surfer you must be true to yourself and others. It may sound corny, but honesty IS the best policy, at least when you deal with me. I aim to own my self-care failures just as firmly as I do my successes. There are not too many problems I can't help people with, but if lies and mistruths become a barrier to good communication, then only superficial actions ever get accomplished.

Lying and misrepresenting is a very dangerous sandbar to the Sugar Surfer. It's challenging to the family working with a budding young surfer. Realize that the sandbar of mistrust will always thwart quality Sugar Surfing. By all means trust... and verify.

Riptides and sandbars are the hazards below the surface which undermine the success of many well intentioned Sugar Surfers and their families. You might think of several others after reading this chapter. Make an effort to keep these sources of self-care error in the back of your mind when troubleshooting and problem-solving your daily Sugar Surfing moves and methods.

This page has been sponsored by: Type 1 Technology Ventures, LLC

Hollow Highs

Chapter 11

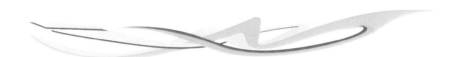

Hollow highs. This is a term I use to explain a high blood sugar caused by stress. The reason I say "hollow" is that many times these high BG surges or spikes don't require as much correction insulin (nudging) compared to a rising or high BG from food, especially food containing lots of carbs. Sometimes these highs will correct themselves in an hour or two without any help. Managing hollow highs requires that you keep your head in the game and actually think about what might be causing each high blood sugar. Every situation is just a bit different so let me outline some common scenarios with the intention of unraveling some of the mystery behind what may seem like just more diabetes 'mumbo-jumbo'.

Example 1 – Sports and Exercise

You or your child with diabetes participates in an intense sports activity. There is often excitement, tension, and maybe a touch of anxiety leading up to the start of the competition or as the event progresses. Watching the CGM readout during the activity or afterwards may show anything from a slow steady rise to a rapid spike in BG that has nothing to do with food or drink. In fact, no food or drinks with carbs may have even been consumed for hours before this happens. Don't forget that many athletes casually consume liquid carbs during an activity to maintain a steady stream of energy for working muscles. Usually this is in the form of different brands of 'sport' or energy drinks.

So what's really happening? The body's response to exercise is largely identical to the response it has to stress. I tend to say that stress is "exercise without the movement". When a sudden physical challenge or threat presents itself, in a very short time the body must get prepared for immediate combat or a rapid withdrawal (run away) from whatever stressful or challenging situation is unfolding before us. This basic human response is part of our survival mechanism against perceived threats, physical obstacles, and predators. You may have heard this response to stress called the "fight or flight" response. Running away from or fighting an adversary consumes lots of energy for muscles and the brain. Blood sugar is the high octane energy source that muscles need to effectively perform those actions. In diabetes, our body's are missing an important element.

Athletes apply this physiologic response to perform incredible feats of prowess or break new endurance records. In diabetes, one very important part of this system is not working the way it should: insulin. In the non-diabetic person, the blood insulin level drops rapidly with exercise. This is due to an insulin "cut-off switch" in the pancreas that originates from the vagus nerve, which comes directly from the brain.

Quickly lowering the insulin supply in the bloodstream allows a non-diabetic person to coordinate the quick drop in insulin levels with a matching increase in other substances (mainly anti-insulin hormones) that together act to raise sugar levels internally. This sugar surge provides the high energy fuel for active muscles. For people with the

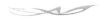

ability to produce insulin, their insulin levels fall just the right amount to allow all this to happen, automatically.

With T1D, if insulin drops too low, then the imbalance between insulin and anti-insulin forces will send you down the path to high blood sugar and DKA. If the insulin levels are not lowered enough, the combined effect of the higher insulin levels together with the exercise may lower the blood sugar levels, resulting in low blood sugar. This can happen even with the anti-insulin hormones present. This is why exercise has such a "wild card" effect on BG levels in persons with type 1 diabetes. It all depends on the balance of insulin relative to the anti-insulin forces in the blood at the time the exercise occurs.

Under normal circumstances, the ability to downshift or reduce insulin levels quickly is necessary for the other "anti-insulin" hormones (the ones that raise sugar levels) to do their jobs properly. The end result is a steady stream of high energy glucose to fuel active muscles, heart and lungs. In persons with diabetes taking insulin by injection or through a pump, it's harder to coordinate a sudden drop in insulin to just the right levels to allow for the right amount of sugar to be released into the blood by the "stress hormones". In many cases, the result is likely to be a low blood sugar, since insulin levels could not be shut down enough and too much insulin along with exercise drops sugar levels.

In other cases, there might actually need to be more insulin needed to counter-balance the BG raising effects of the anticipated exercise or unexpected stressful event. I tend to see more unexplained high BG levels in athletes who play sports with longer periods of inactivity. This includes sports that depend on high energy spurts with periods of inactivity, even standing (like in an outfielder in baseball or sitting on the bench during the game). Sports where there seems to be constant motion (e.g., soccer, tennis, and basketball) seem more prone to low BG if precautions are not taken. These are my general observations.

The bottom line here: Exercise will have variable effects on most persons with type 1 diabetes. The best approach is to expect this variability and learn to Sugar Surf through these events with the least amount of turbulence. Most of all, avoid the wipeout.

Example 2 – School Stress

A boy with type 1 diabetes and severe dyslexia (a learning disability which makes reading a challenge) is starting 5th grade. Prior to school his BG tracings on his CGM were well managed. But on the days he attends school he gets a huge BG spike in the morning. These spikes are not seen on days he is not in class. His eating habits are the same on school and non-school days as is his usual level of activity in the mornings. So what's going on? Stress. In 5th grade there is a greater emphasis on reading and reporting on what was read. Due to his severe reading problem, this created tremendous emotional stress which acted to drive his blood sugar levels up. His body was essentially preparing him to run away or fight, but that response was not an option.

With time and some academic help, his blood sugars improved. Even without treatment, his BG levels usually returned to in range levels by late morning so the family chose not to correct them. The class that stressed him was only an hour long so the pressure on his sugar level ended and his BG levels drifted back down to in range levels.

Had they corrected him with insulin, the results could have been scattered. A full "correction" dose of insulin given at the peak of the high BG might have been too much, and would have dropped him low by lunchtime or afterwards. In these situations, it's best to watch and see what consistent pattern emerges before stepping in too aggressively with corrections. In fact the first impression most people would make was that this was a food problem. With a few more questions we were able to rule this out.

In this case a little time, patience, and tutoring actually helped correct the BG problem. The boy's mid-morning BG spikes improved within a month or two as his reading skills improved and changes in

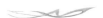

his individualized learning plan were implemented. The parents might have tried different foods for breakfast but that probably would not have worked very well since stress induced hyperglycemia is not food driven as I explain further on.

Example 3 – Situational Stress

Here is another example of a long term stressful situation as seen through the eyes of my CGM.

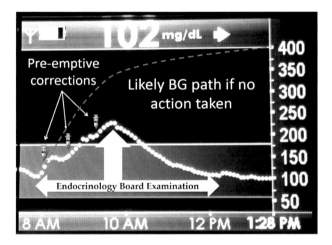

I am required to take a major written examination to remain certified in my medical specialty of endocrinology. Fortunately this exam is only once every 10 years. It's long, grueling, and very stressful. You can see my BG response to this and how I tackled it with injections to try and balance my rapid acting insulin against the stress hormones coursing through my veins acting to drive up my sugar levels. Once the exam was over and the stress was gone, I had to be watchful that I didn't fall low due to one of the later doses of insulin. It's always important to be watchful of the CGM readout during the hours after a meal time or correction insulin dose. Glances are usually enough. And yes, I passed my exam!

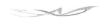

Example 4 – Short Term Stress

One of my practice partners also has type 1 diabetes and also wears a sensor. Here is a side by side image of our CGM readouts during a departmental staff meeting.

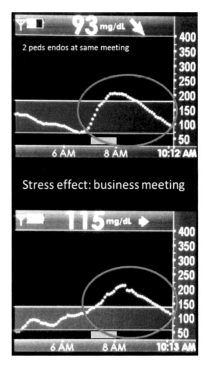

In this monthly meeting, we often listen to distressing information about "how things are changing" (e.g. - pay structure, retirement benefits and duty hours, etc...) based on the ongoing changes in 21st century medical practices. We both quietly sat there but our inner emotions expressed themselves in these surges of blood sugar. Thankfully the meeting is only one hour long and afterwards the readings usually drift down over a few hours, but in both cases we took a smaller than usual correction dose of rapid-acting insulin to bring the BG down a bit sooner. I could have waited another couple of hours and seen if it would come down on its own, but we both chose to take a small correction (about 50% of what I would otherwise take for that level in a non-stressful situation). You can see what happened next.

Origin of a "Hollow High"

All these examples illustrate different ways that BG can surge in the absence of extra food. Hollow Highs are just as real as any other high BG level. It's the force behind the high that's different. Since there is less "substance" to the rising blood sugar, it typically requires less downward force (insulin, or even exercise) to move or manipulate the trend downward towards your target range as compared to a rising BG

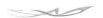

created by food or drink from a meal or snack.

Sugar is constantly entering and leaving the bloodstream one second to the next. The representation of this phenomenon along a BG dot-line is what I've described earlier as flux and drift. That's the end result we see on the sensor. Sugar Surfers know more than just the number. We know the what, the why and the how that helps us to manage our diabetes rather than letting it manage us.

Under normal conditions the adult liver stores around 75 grams of carbohydrates. Among the many wonderful things the liver does, it sustains blood sugar levels between meals and during long periods of time without eating (like overnight or fasting). It does that by being an organ that both stores and releases sugar, much like the battery in my hybrid car stores electricity and uses it to keep the motor turning at a steady speed. The muscles also contain a smaller amount of carbs, as do the kidneys. But for the sake of this discussion I focus only on the role of our liver.

If you have ever used the injectable hormone glucagon to treat a severe low blood sugar, what you're doing is triggering a hormonal surge (glucagon is a hormone, it's not a form sugar) aimed at the liver to tell it to "dump" or release some of its supply of stored sugar directly into the bloodstream as soon as possible.

Just like rapid-acting insulin, glucagon takes 15-20 minutes after an injection to raise the blood sugar. A full dose glucagon injection (1 mg) will usually raise the BG rather high over the next couple of hours and might even cause nausea as a side effect (glucagon is a gut hormone and a brain hormone). In essence, glucagon releases a "sugar tsunami" from the liver that washes through the system. Like rapid-acting insulin, glucagon's effect does not persist very long.

Anyone with diabetes who has ever gotten an epinephrine shot for an allergic reaction or severe asthma attack will see a similar effect since epinephrine (adrenaline) is also a rapid acting stress hormone. Once the effect of the short acting glucagon (or epinephrine) passes, there is no

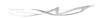

further force to drive more sugar into the bloodstream. Other stress hormones, including cortisol and growth hormone, have a slower and longer lasting effect of raising BG levels which lasts for hours and perhaps longer.

As I said, stress is exercise without the movement. Physical actions contribute to getting rid of excess blood sugar during exercise or sports by busy muscles. Unfortunately, sitting still in a classroom or a board meeting doesn't offer easy alternatives to burning off all that excess sugar that was unknowingly dumped into the blood stream. So, our sugar levels tend to be at the mercy of whatever insulin level is present in our systems when these events occur. The simple act of wearing a CGM allows us to see this effect as it happens unlike the experience of only using a blood sugar meter. Beyond seeing real-time dots and numbers, Sugar Surfing is a method that allows us to better understand what these dots and numbers mean and how to best manage so many different situations.

Many of us get confused about how exercise or stress can have different effects from day to day on blood sugars trends. The only thing constant about how stress affects blood sugar levels in diabetes is that it is always inconsistent.

Managing a "Hollow High"

Pay attention to what stress does to your BG profile and watch it over time so you can create a profile or inventory of your unique responses to stress. Experiencing a few high BG episodes as you define a particular stressful event's effect will not have any harmful long term consequences. Try to find patterns in your behaviors that seem to occur predictably from day to day which cause these highs to happen. I suppose I could choose to skip stressful meetings, I can sometimes do that, but longer term I need to learn how to manage my stress and my diabetes. Try different types of stress management techniques like yoga, go for a run, listen to relaxing music or take a nap if you can swing it.

Use basic Sugar Surfing principles to manage Hollow Highs. I started by correcting these highs with less insulin (50% less than what I normally use for a non-stress-induced high BG consistently works best for me). Careful experimenting with close glancing of my CGM readout allowed me to experiment with smaller insulin doses (nudges) to accomplish this with less chance of overshooting my desired BG target range a few hours later.

I now pre-empt these highs with that same corrective dose (50%), but now I take these in advance of the high, delivered as I see the rising BG trend cross my upper "action threshold" of 140 mg/dL (7.8 mmol/L).

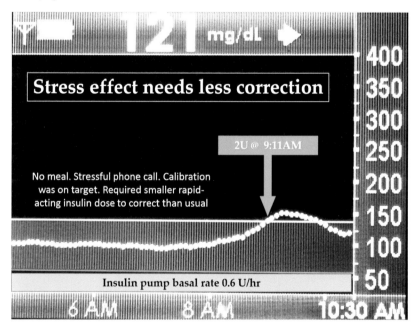

Discover what you consistently do that seems to be associated with stress highs and make mental (or better yet written) notes of it. Also understand that as you attempt to control or manipulate your Hollow Highs with insulin or exercise your results will be scattered and inconsistent at first. Like with other surfing skills, don't give up after

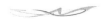

the first several attempts. Lots of pivoting might be needed. You may fail at first. However, successful Sugar Surfing requires that you learn from earlier failed attempts and commit to make the next effort better.

Organized sporting events are by their very nature more predictable, at least in regards to timing. Spontaneous activities are more chaotic. Patterns can be uncovered in either situation. Scheduled meetings or classes are predictable. Being called to the principal's office, getting into a verbal argument or fight, getting stuck in bumper to bumper traffic, dissolving a close relationship, or getting a speeding ticket are part of the fabric of life and each of these will push our BG trends in different directions.

Sugar Surfing is about finding ways to keep your head in the game when these kinds of events seek to knock you off your board. When they say you'd better bring your "A-game" I like to think the A stands for Attitude. Sugar Surfers have a great attitude toward mastering their diabetes. You can, too. Push through adversity and don't get discouraged when life throws you a curve. Just learn how to bank through it. Glance at your CGM, verify with your meter and apply your well-practiced Sugar Surfing skills.

Now that you know that all highs are not created equal it's your responsibility to:

- ○ Identify a Hollow High; and,

- ○ Take a different course of action as compared to a post meal high, for example.

Surf Safely

Chapter 12

Insulin is a Sugar Surfer's most potent weapon. It demands the utmost respect and must be properly cared for and maintained. Proper insulin storage and care are the responsibility of the person taking insulin or their family. Extremes of heat and cold will damage insulin, as will violent shaking or prolonged exposure to sunlight. Treat insulin as you would treat eggs.

Sugar Surfing requires an understanding of how your insulin works after an injection. There are four properties of all injected insulin preparations that you should become familiar with: 1) Onset of action; 2) Peak activity; 3) Duration of action; and, 4) Inconsistency.

Onset of action

The time from when an insulin injection is given to when the insulin has a detectable effect on lowering BG levels is the insulin's onset of action. Onset of insulin action varies based on the type of insulin, amount given and even the site of the injection. Rapid-acting insulins (insulin lispro, insulin aspart and insulin glulisine) usually start to lower BG levels in 15-20 minutes. Long-acting insulin (insulin glargine, insulin detemir) takes two to four hours before showing any effect on BG levels.

Peak activity

The time when an injected insulin dose exerts its maximum blood sugar lowering effect is called its peak. Usually this is more of a range than it is a specific point in time. Like the eye of a hurricane, the peak effect slowly passes, but remember that larger insulin doses generally have longer peak duration compared to smaller doses. Most rapid acting insulin preparations peak between 45 - 90 minutes. Long acting insulin preparations are not supposed to show any peak activity but recent studies have shown that in some patients, definite peaks activity do exist contrary to what we've all be taught.

Duration of action

An insulin dose eventually loses its sugar lowering effect as the body breaks it down and removes it from the blood stream. The range of time required for this removal process is known as the duration of insulin action. It's usually measured in hours. Insulin duration will also change based on the size of the insulin dose taken, type of insulin, and the ability of the body to remove it. The ability of rapid-acting insulin to lower BG may last anywhere from 2 to 8 hours. Usually, this range is somewhere in-between. Long-acting insulin can last 18 - 30 hours depending on type and amount, plus other factors.

Inconsistency

One quality of insulin that's not well appreciated is its lack of day to day consistency. In fact, the body can react differently to the same injected insulin dose based on time of day, stress, food eaten, amount injected, or site of insulin injection. This irregular response is not

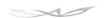

necessarily bad. It's actually part of how a body adapts to changing life circumstances. Plus, as was discussed earlier, "direction affects correction". In other words, a rising or falling BG trend will create different BG results to a dose of rapid-acting insulin no matter how carefully the dose is calculated. Exercise and stress will also influence the effect of an identical dose of insulin from one day to the next. All this variability and inconsistency creates a special challenge to predict insulin's blood sugar lowering action from day to day, which challenges the static model of diabetes care we are usually taught. It's a great argument for the need to Sugar Surf.

In summary, injected insulin has many innate qualities that make it unpredictable. When improper dosing technique, incorrect dosing and omission of insulin doses are factored in, it should be no surprise that insulin is not always the precision tool we are often led to believe.

Other elements of Safe Surfing include the topics discussed on the following pages. They are as important as understanding how your insulin works and require an equal attention to detail.

Insulin dose timing

In spite of all its shortcomings, timing is everything where insulin dosing is concerned. It is part of the rationale behind "Waiting for the Bend" (Chapter 7 – Basic Concepts of Sugar Surfing). Following an injection, rapid acting insulin is absorbed from the injection site by the bloodstream and whisked away to be taken to all body tissues. Before insulin can even reach its target, a large portion of it is destroyed by the liver. Once insulin reaches its target tissues, it then takes time to exert its action on cells to induce them to absorb sugar and start lowering the sugar level in the entire bloodstream. This is why injecting insulin before your meal and waiting for the bend is so often necessary and effective in maintaining post meal BG control.

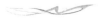

Lag time

The Sugar Surfer must grasp the concept of sensor lag time in order to make important decisions in regards to insulin dosing. As sugar levels change in blood, this is also reflected in the sugar levels in the tissues outside the bloodstream. It also takes several minutes for sugar levels in blood to stabilize in the tissues where a glucose sensor is placed.

Because of lag time, current CGM sensors reflect blood sugar levels that are up to 12 to 20 minutes old. When blood sugar levels are trending steady, these devices are more likely to show BG results which are closer to the actual level in the blood at that moment. If BG levels are changing rapidly, there is a greater likelihood of a meaningful discrepancy between the blood and tissue BG levels. This fact is useful to know in cases where treatment has been given for a low BG level, the person's symptoms are obviously improving and the sensor screen still reads low.

When rapid-acting insulin is taken, there is another lag time to consider; the onset of insulin action described earlier. This means that when you "Wait for the Bend" you are waiting for the insulin to get delivered to body tissues and to begin lowering sugar levels. Don't forget about that lag time... we also have to wait several minutes before the sensor is able to detect the change in blood sugar via the interstitial fluids of the body which bathe the cells. Where insulin action is concerned, it's the sum of several different individual lag times that all contribute to the number displayed on your receiver.

To be clear, there are two lag times to understand. The first is the insulin action lag time described above. Second is the sensor detection lag time. As faster acting insulins are created, the combined sensor lag will get shorter when measuring the effect of an insulin dose. The speed at which blood sugar equalizes within the interstitial fluid (where all commercially available sensors measures sugar) will always result in a significant delay or lag. There are other sensor technologies which

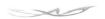

measure glucose differently and which may be able to shorten that lag time but for now they are involved in research studies. So, until we can measure blood sugar directly in real-time, there will always be some amount of lag time that must be considered and appreciated. Surfers must become comfortable with factoring time and other variables into their decision making. This is not unlike how ocean surfers must time their entry onto an emerging wave.

Sugar Surfers appreciate the irregular nature of insulin action. They are not surprised by it. Good surfers are always willing to make changes in their routine to adapt to its ways. Most of all, they aim to manipulate insulin to best suit their needs within the limitations of their particular CGM system.

Meter use

CGM devices provide only estimates of the blood sugar. At times, a sensor might be so well calibrated that it matches the finger stick BG perfectly. Yet at other times these results might be very far apart. There are excellent methods to maximize sensor calibration (see Chapter 6 – Waxing your Board). The truth is that with so many variables in play and that these devices are measuring different things, it is merely a coincidence if the numbers match or are very close to each other. The odds of them matching are not in their favor and they are not designed to match. They need to be in the same neighborhood but matching up should not be your expectation.

The good Sugar Surfer should verify with their BG meter when making a treatment decision based on a trending BG reading on a sensor. This meter reading can also be used to add an additional calibration point too. Please do not use every meter BG reading for calibration purposes. If you suspect you know the reason for a large difference between your CGM and your meter's BG reading (flux, for example) then wait a while for things to settle down and re-check. However, if you don't have any reason to believe there could be a large difference then go ahead and use the meter reading to calibrate the

sensor. It usually helps.

As discussed in Chapter 5 - False Idols, BG meters are always a potential source of error, too. For now, BG meters are still considered more accurate than sensor data. The greatest advantage of the CGM is its ability to conveniently reveal trending patterns.

Stacking insulin

There is a "sacred cow" of type 1 diabetes care: insulin stacking. The simplest definition of 'stacking' is to take a rapid acting insulin dose while another previous dose is still working thus causing an overlap in the insulin effects. This term is generally intended to apply to rapid-acting doses only, although it is feasible to overlap basal insulin (long lasting insulin) doses if the doses are large enough.

The problem with insulin stacking happens when doses of insulin are injected (or infused from a pump) closely together in time without awareness of blood sugar level and the amount of residual bolus insulin on board. Hence, insulin effects from any additional doses will overlap with each other making it more likely for severe low blood sugar (hypoglycemia) to occur. Insulin stacking should only be considered when there is awareness of the BG and residual insulin; a skill that can be mastered.

Technically speaking, persons with diabetes are stacking insulin all the time. Basal insulin (whether by pump or injection) acts as a floor upon which rapid acting insulin works. Since the BG lowering effect of long acting insulin (or a properly set insulin pump basal rate) is minimal, the main BG lowering usually comes from the rapid-acting insulin. Exercise can also lower BG and can magnify the stacking effect of any insulin dose.

The major consequence of insulin stacking is referred to in regards to doses taken to correct high blood sugar readings. In these situations, if more than one correction dose is given due to the lack of any apparent BG lowering effect, the general concern is that the

overlapping of these doses with a second dose may cause low blood sugar. In the days when most patients only check blood sugar four times per day this is absolutely a warranted precaution. The term insulin stacking was coined years before the era of continuous glucose monitoring.

In those days, the direction of glucose trends was difficult to easily measure without high frequency blood sugar monitoring. It is common sense to think that overlapping insulin doses would create more risks than benefits to most persons with diabetes. For these reasons the concept of using overlapping rapid acting insulin doses has been actively discouraged. Some doctors forbid taking insulin between meals, even for corrections. In those cases, the correction can only be taken at mealtime.

With Sugar Surfing, people are much more aware of their situation and will not hesitate to verify high risk blood sugar situations with a finger-stick, a test strip and your meter. Continuous glucose monitoring changes the old ways, at least for some. For example, the bi-hormonal artificial pancreas (currently in development) relies on controlled insulin stacking algorithms to attain near normal blood sugar levels in its users. But the AP also has the ability to counteract the effect of overshooting the target blood sugar mark by its ability to also deliver a blood sugar raising substance: glucagon. This is similar to how the non-diabetic body maintains in-range blood sugar levels.

Stacking insulin is allowed by insulin pumps using bolus calculators, but with modifications. Based on the pump's pre-programmed duration of insulin value, a rapid-acting insulin dose used for a high BG correction can be reduced by an amount which is estimated by the pump (and even some mobile apps) to be active or still working. The pump calculates the estimated remaining insulin action from a prior bolus, by considering the current blood sugar measurement entered, and then subtracting the remaining active insulin to give its recommendation. It's all based on a mathematical formula and does not consider or factor in any awareness of the BG

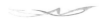

direction or trend. Unfortunately many people don't routinely check BG before dosing and many don't use their bolus calculators, raising the risk for unintentional insulin stacking. To make matters worse, not all pumps use the same mathematical equation. Sadly, some insulin pumps consider active residual meal bolus insulin whereas others do not. Be sure that you know exactly how your pump 'wizard' works and in great detail. Just reference your user manual or call the manufacturer's support phone number or website.

It's time to take another look at taking rapid acting insulin doses delivered closer together than previously recommended. Since CGM technology allows the opportunity to visualize blood sugar trends and directions, more aggressive insulin and carbohydrate therapy is possible to manage a trending BG pattern in either direction. I believe careful insulin stacking with modifications can be a valid approach to diabetes care under the right circumstances. To be clear, this requires vigilance and preparation to perform properly and is a very advanced Sugar Surfing tactic. Never bolus indiscriminately without thinking through the situation!

Advice and tips for overlapping rapid-acting insulin doses

Let me remind you of some basic Sugar Surfing techniques that are always available to you. The more you use these basic maneuvers the less likely you are going to find yourself in a situation that might tempt you to employ the advanced and risky move of stacking insulin doses. Just know that balancing insulin and food is an inexact science and adjustments with follow-up are often needed. Here's how it's done.

At a scheduled meal, take the mealtime dose in advance of the meal and "Wait for the Bend" as discussed in earlier chapters. This assumes the meal is not low carb or slow carb and that you're not already starting with a low blood sugar. In those cases a different dosing strategy is needed. Watching trend lines and deciding when to eat requires a working understanding of the food you are eating and the speed that it converts to sugar in your system, under most

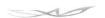

circumstances. I have a personal list of favorite meals that I've learned over time to have fast, medium or slow speeds of conversion to sugar after I finish eating them. Doing my homework is part of good Sugar Surfing. My first attempt at timing insulin for a new meal or food might fail. If it does, and I like that food, then I will try a different dosing strategy next time. It might be timing based or I might need to use the combination or extended bolus feature on my insulin pump. If I'm not wearing a pump I will use the "I-chains" method described in Chapter 14 - Surfing Rail to Rail. Like a good surfer, I pick the right board for the surf I'm heading into. It always makes for a smoother ride.

Next, watch the BG trend line frequently after the insulin and the meal. Set an upper BG limit or threshold at which time you would consider taking an additional dose. Choosing a relatively high threshold when first learning this skill is wise. For example, select 250 mg/dL (13.9 mmol/L) as a trigger to consider taking a supplemental insulin dose. Check your BG to verify and then calculate the amount of insulin that you think should be needed to lower the reading back to your desired target BG (120 mg/dL [6.7 mmol/L], for example).

You should not attempt overlapping insulin effects like this until you have learned to micro-bolus. The ideal starting dose should be calculated with your pump's bolus calculator factoring in the BG level. Based on the duration of insulin action factor already in your pump (and hopefully activated), the pump will suggest a correction dose that is modified by the amount of insulin it "thinks" is still active and remaining in your body. Remember, each pump manufacturer has different ways of counting what is active so you need to verify with your pump manufacturer. Don't assume! Chances are that the dose is not sufficient, but for teaching purposes use this dose anyway.

After that dose is taken, wait and watch your CGM readout often. It might take up to 3 hours to see the final results. I suggest glancing every 15 minutes. Find your own glancing frequency. I hyper-glance in the time leading up to and immediately after finishing my meals. This allows me to catch the earliest sign of a possible inflection of the trend

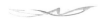

line that might suggest the need for more food (carbs) or even a pre-emptive dose of insulin (see Rail to Rail surfing). This is especially important if I think a special treat may be in my immediate future. Planning ahead often allows me to be in the right spot to enjoy the occasional guilt-free high carb meal, snack or dessert. That's living a normal life at least in my book and it's what I aim to do for myself and what I advise my patients to strive for.

What your first attempt may show is a turning of the trend line as a result of the extra insulin dose. The BG trend should ideally slowly curve around and track back towards your BG target range. If your basal rate is set properly (see Chapter 7) the trend line will start to 'level out' near your target BG within 30 mg/dL (1.7 mmol/L rounded to 2) in either direction. This is what you practice for over and over. Repetition is key.

If you look to be overshooting your BG target range and heading for a low BG, then preselect an action threshold in the other direction to eat a "braking dose" of fast-acting carbohydrates. A good starting point is 15 grams. The rate of drop will dictate when to treat a falling low. If BG is falling fast, then treating at a sensor readout of 150 mg/dL (8.3 mmol/L) would seem proper because a meter check done then would be lower than the sensor read-out due to sensor lag time. If the BG drop is more gradual, then holding off on eating a fast acting braking carbohydrate would be proper at least until below 80 mg/dL (4.4 mmol/L). And the amount of braking carbs might be less based on the rate of fall. In general, if your downward speed is angled, you can often wait and watch for leveling out to occur. If that does not appear to be happening, then select a treatment threshold about 10 - 20 mg/dL (0.6 – 1.1 mmol/L) higher than your low alert and treat with fast acting carbs at that time. If you are young or prone to rapid drops, set your action threshold for treating with carbs at a higher level in order to catch your plummeting lows early.

You need to create a range of insulin doses that you know will lower your BG levels from your action threshold dose (in this case, 250

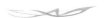

mg/dL [13.9 mmol/L]) back towards the middle of your target range. Aim higher at first, such as 150 mg/dL (8.3 mmol/L). Hitting your zone would be seen as a leveled off trend line between 120 and 180 mg/dL (6.7 – 10 mmol/L). As your skills improve, you can start to consider lowering your target zone and mid-point. Don't rush things. It took me a couple of years to map out all my own responses.

Insulin stacking at night

Generally, I do not recommend that you take overlapping insulin doses during sleeping hours. In general, persons are more sensitive to insulin in the overnight hours than during the day. And a "low" CGM alarm may be missed or ignored if you (and/or your sleep partner) are in a deep sleep, increasing the risk of an unexpected severe low BG.

One special exception is what I call the "sleep bolus" which I created several years ago at diabetes camp. We found that correcting a high BG at bedtime using an extended/square wave bolus was possible and effective. For an extra safety buffer, we programmed the pump to deliver 50% - 70% of the normal calculated correction dose over 5 - 6 hours instead of all at once. This maneuver gradually returns the BG closer to baseline with lower risk of middle of the night low blood sugar. To be safe at first, practice sleep bolusing during the day and make sure you monitor BG through the night until you are comfortable with the method and the results you observe.

Caveats of stacking

Insulin 'stacking' can be a valid approach to diabetes care under controlled circumstances. Safe stacking is possible only if the person or family is committed to being hyper vigilant with BG checks or CGM glancing for many hours after two closely spaced doses of rapid-acting insulin are taken. Don't stack at night or when asleep. It invites problems. Stacking examples will be described in Chapter 14 referred to in the context of taking insulin to "pre-empt" a rising BG level.

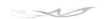

Always be prepared and vigilant!

I use fast acting carbs to nudge my BG trend line through the day and at night as needed. That means I keep carbs within my reach at all times. I keep glucose tablets and juice (grape is my favorite) on my nightstand for any trending lows at night. My car has the same items in the pockets by my seat. I also keep carbs on hand at the office and glucose tabs in my coat pocket or backpack. When I travel, I have glucose tabs on the plane in my coat pocket or personal carry-on items. I'm always prepared. I call this move "Sugar Stashing".

The same preparation applies to insulin. When I wear my pump I always have insulin pens as a backup in case of a pump or site malfunction. When I travel I keep my insulin with me on the plane at all times. I can and will Sugar Surf anywhere. It's not only my right… it's the right thing to do so don't let anyone put a crimp in what you need to do or how you decide to do it.

My BG meter, strips and lancets are also part of my basic self-care toolkit. These items are also always on my person or easily within reach.

Be careful when putting on or removing tight clothing since a sensor can become dislodged during these common daytime activities. When bathing or showering I always protect the sensor site from prolonged exposure to water, since it could result in detachment. I'm spatially aware of my sensor location. This has kept me from knocking off the sensor in a door jam, getting into and out of my small car, wearing a seat belt, playing high impact sports, and even just sitting in a crowded airline seat.

Develop your own surf colony

Surfing is something only one person can do fully, but it sure helps to have your own surf colony supporting you. Your team may consist of loved ones, close friends, and your diabetes provider. It's also more fun to include your team on your surfing adventures, especially if you

are part of a family. I see surfing as a team sport.

Type 1 diabetes has always been a self-managed disease. Hundreds of choices are made every day which shape the speed and direction of the energy that flows through our bodies. If we are to Surf Safely, we must know and appreciate the strengths and weaknesses of our tools, especially insulin. We must be prepared for the unexpected, and if we fail, then fail safe. Surfers gain wisdom from missteps and are willing to take on new challenges without fear of failure. Teamwork and communication are hallmarks of responsible Sugar Surfers.

Like any method, Sugar Surfing is no better or worse than the person applying it. In poorly prepared hands, glycemic wipeouts will be more common than "in the zone" BG trends. The theme of this chapter is to always have the safety of the person or child with diabetes in mind. Safe Surfing also means being prepared for the unexpected. It demands ongoing attention to detail and consistency. Its ultimate goal is to improve daily diabetes self-management and enhance personal confidence in one's decision making abilities as they relate to daily dynamic diabetes management in the moment.

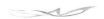

A Day of Surfing

Chapter 13

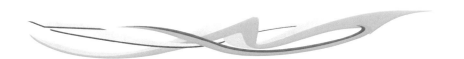

To put these concepts together in a really definitive way I have assembled this Chapter to show you how one single day in my life occurred through the lens of Sugar Surfing. Each image is annotated and explained.

Now that you are familiar with the basic Sugar Surfing concepts and moves, you will recognize them in these slides and be able to see them in action.

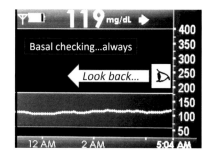

First things first: wake up, look back. This is the most basic Sugar Surfing maneuver. On this day there were slow BG drifts to adjust. No drops or spikes during the night. I aim for 100 mg/dL (5.6 mmol/L) when I awaken. For me this straight line trend is slightly high. For others this might be just fine. That's your decision. At 9pm the prior evening, I had taken 18 units of insulin glargine (Lantus). My basal insulin was doing its job this day.

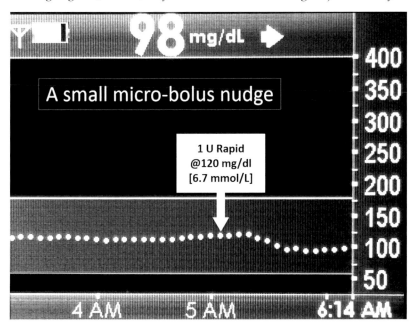

My morning calibration BG this day was in agreement at 120 mg/dL (6.7 mmol/L). I chose to microbolus 1 unit of insulin aspart (Novolog) at 5:07 am. I knew from prior experience and practice that I would drift down about 20-30 mg/dL (1-1.6 mmol/L) in the next one to two hours. You can see the lag and the slow drift downward on the right. I'm not advocating this, but I show it to make a point about how these trends can be gently steered under the right conditions. Insulin responses differ between people and must be individualized.

I eat a similar meal most work day mornings as a matter of habit. I've learned its glycemic profile and know how to time my insulin in advance. So at 6:29 am., I injected 3 units insulin aspart (Novolog) and started to wait for the bend as I went about my morning routine.

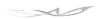

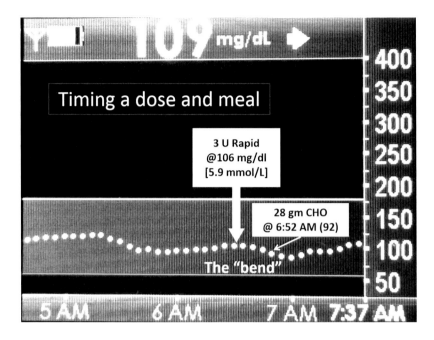

No correction insulin was needed since I had taken it earlier after waking up. As the BG trend dots began to shift downward, I could sense this. I then ate my already prepared breakfast. It's important to note the lack of an after meal BG spike or rise in the two hours following breakfast. Over time, after meal BG responses like this act as a significant lowering effect to my A1C. My meter BG read 92 mg/dL (5.1 mmol/L) when I ate which was another way I proved my insulin was working based on the prior reading of 106 mg/dL (5.9 mmol/L).

After arriving at work, a hectic day at the clinic ensued. I experienced a slow upward BG trend from 7:00 to 8:00 (red arrow). I check my BG (126 mg/dL; 7 mmol/L). Rather than having it go higher, I chose to take 2 units insulin aspart. But this was more likely a "hollow high" due to morning work stress and a full work schedule. After the pivot that followed, I started a BG drop that seemed to be going further than I wanted it to go.

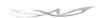

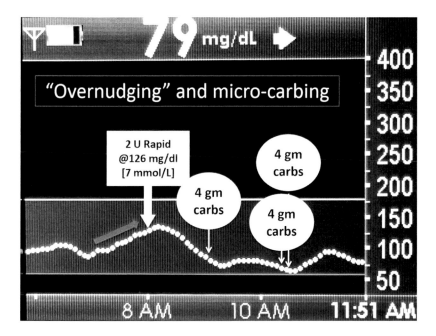

So at 9:19 am, I chose to micro-carb 4 grams of glucose (1 tab) to slow down the drop and level out my BG dot line. As I zipped in and out of exam rooms, I started noticing small BG dips. Looking back, I likely over treated the 8 am rise with the 2 unit bolus and should have waited longer or taken less insulin to slow down the rise. In total, I took 12 grams of extra carbs over the next couple of hours to offset downward BG drifts. I was never outwardly symptomatic with a low but I could "sense" the drifts.

By lunch, I'm seeing a slightly downward BG drift again. I injected 1 unit less insulin this time as compared to my usual lunch time dose. As I was already drifting very gradually downward, I chose to eat my meal a little sooner since there was less need to "Wait for the Bend".

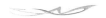

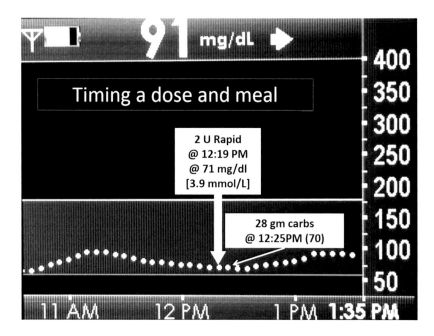

You can see a slight later BG rise which never quite rose above 100 mg/dL (5.6 mmol/L). Recall that non-diabetic BG levels remain under 140 mg/dL (7.8 mmol/L) two hours after completing a standard carbohydrate meal load. I'm meeting and exceeding that expectation as seen in the image above.

As the afternoon progressed, I felt some very subtle downward drifts. Because I'm in the moment, I checked my BG and micro-carbed a couple of times with 4 gram glucose tablets to raise my BG level up, but not too much.

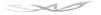

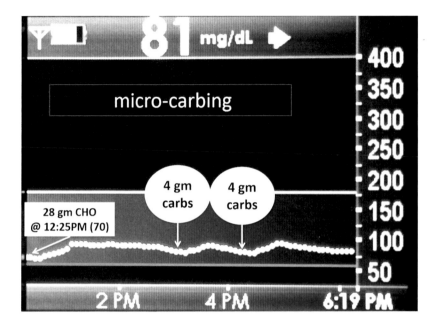

If I wanted to create an illustration for "micro-pivoting", I suppose this would be it. Sugar Surfing has enough terminology already.

Later that evening, my family and I chose to go to a local Japanese restaurant. I selected the soft shell crab, something I eat infrequently and never before at this particular location. Before dinner (and not really knowing what I was going to order) I took an injection of insulin aspart at 7:51 pm to offset a rising BG trend that started at 7:00 pm. At this point I'm glancing more often at my sensor and will continue to pay closer attention through the meal as I always do.

I will also glance at my CGM readout often over the next couple of hours. Fifteen minutes later I ordered my meal. I took what I felt would be a proper starting dose of insulin aspart (6 units) for what I thought I would be eating. There were ample carbs served with the meal but I was not planning to consume a lot of rice which I know from previous experience really spikes my blood sugars. I knew the breading on some of the fried appetizers would cause a later rise in my BG as many fried

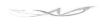

and battered foods tend to do.

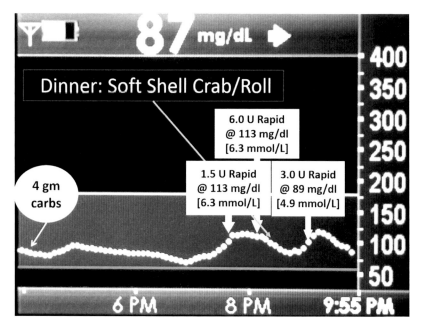

In fact there was a drop afterwards, but nothing went too low as you can see. A late rise that I was anticipating began around 9:00 pm. I attributed this in part to the fried appetizers and only because I was paying attention was I able to take a preemptive dose to cover this late rise.

My after dinner BG levels stabilized sufficiently that at 10:22 pm I was in a suitable range to get to sleep. Again, this is according to my own comfort zone and personal experiences. You might have made a different decision and you wouldn't necessarily have been wrong. The overnight tracing that followed looked a lot like the one that started the day before. Looking at this 24 hour tracing, notice that this is in essence a non-diabetic BG trend line.

This is about as good as it gets. A very important teaching point: I will never again have a 24 hour tracing that looks exactly like this. Each day truly is unique from a blood sugar point of view.

Diabetes control always exists "in the moment". It is not something that is written out completely in advance, it is not just about taking an insulin dose, checking a BG reading or eating a certain amount of food and it can't be dispensed by one person to another. Diabetes control is the sum

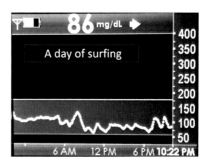

of hundreds of decisions we must make each day. These images aim to highlight a few of those choices and why they were made. It also points out mistakes that can be made and how to recover from them.

Sugar Surfers embrace this proactive-reactive philosophy; the Yin and the Yang of Sugar Surfing. Learn from it, move on and prepare to take on the next wave.

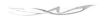

Surfing Rail to Rail

Chapter 14

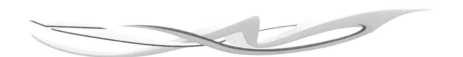

According to SurfScience.com, "Rail to Rail" ocean surfing means riding on your surfboard with your rail (one edge of the board) in the water. This is mainly done on high performance short board surfboards that slow down when they are going straight but speed up when turning 'on a rail'. If you ever watch a pro surfer, they're constantly turning or pumping quickly from side to side. This is rail to rail surfing. Rail to Rail Sugar Surfing is about taking ownership of your diabetes in every way possible. Pivoting is the Sugar Surfing term I created that describes the rail to rail concept.

Pivoting

Pivoting is the essence of Sugar Surfing. It's the action of turning or steering BG trends using a CGM as a real time compass combined with prudent use of your BG meter for verification.

I'm using this previously shared image to illustrate the concept. Notice that the yellow arrows show "elbows" in the 24 hour trend line. Each elbow represents Sugar Surfing methods applied to change the direction of a trending BG level. This book has introduced you to many

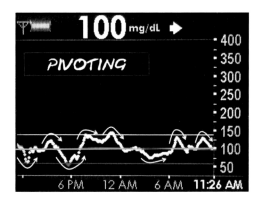

methods to steer a BG trend. Pivoting is the expression of these tools in the form of numerous personal choices, actions and reassessments. When done as a seamless continuum, you direct the trend line where you want it to go.

Throughout this chapter you will see many examples of pivoting in action. You start by having a target to aim at. This can be a specific BG number target that you might already have or it could be expressed as a BG range with upper and lower BG numbers defining the range. I actually use both but select a point at the center of my range as my fulcrum or "pivot point". Like the North Star serving as a fixed reference point to navigate by, I use my pivot point or range in every decision I make about my diabetes.

Micro-dosing

This brings us to the next major principle of Sugar Surfing: micro-dosing. Much of what we teach and have been taught about diabetes care amounts to a one size fits all approach: the static thinking that I discussed in earlier chapters. In the pre-sensor era this rationale made sense. But our current philosophy about diabetes management is all about individualized care. Fortunately, Sugar Surfing is the embodiment of that philosophy. Unfortunately, the medical profession doesn't have the resources or funding to teach all persons with diabetes to be experts in all aspects of their own care. I don't like saying this, but

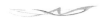

it's true. In spite of our systematic shortcomings, many persons rise above these barriers and find ways to master their diabetes. Many of those accomplished individuals and their families are the supporters and readers of this book.

Once I studied my BG trend patterns and set reasonable alert thresholds, I asked myself a basic question: can I "steer" the path of my blood sugar trend line between meals or scheduled insulin doses? The answer is, "Yes". However, more background is needed first.

Like many others I was taught that if I only could learn to count carbs well enough, checked my BG often, and took the right amount of insulin when I ate, always corrected high and low blood sugars whenever I found them, then my blood sugars should stay in control. I was supposed to keep my blood sugar within a range they called 'normal'. It was pretty standard stuff. On the surface it all sounds easy, right? But much is left out of this oversimplified way of approaching a highly complex problem. It's far fetched to think one can act only a handful of times each day and expect anything but mediocre results. "But I went low carb…and my blood sugar is now easy to manage" you say. That may be, but the ACT of adhering to a low carb diet requires a significant commitment involving many choices per day. If low carb works for you then I'm all for it but most of all I want people to live a happy life and only you can know what that means for you.

By now you've rejected the idea of straight line blood sugar levels all day long, right? Not even non-diabetic persons possess that level of control. There is just way too much variability in all our diabetes devices, insulin, food, and activity. Plus, we're not by our very nature precise and accurate beings. That's just life, in my opinion. So why drag into the discussion of diabetes so much scary talk about exact numbers, obsessing about counting carbs, rigid adherence to exercising regularly, managing stress and illness well, and then bake it in a big pan of fear, blame and guilt to hold it all together?

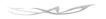

The image below shows how to micro-bolus. It's a small dose of rapid acting insulin taken on a steady BG trend (dot) line. The intent is to move the trend line down and reset into another range. Effective micro-bolusing assumes the basal insulin is properly set. Each Sugar Surfing principle is built on a foundation of other principles. In this example, a small dose of rapid acting insulin is taken as BG levels are trending steady. BG is 120 mg/dL (6.7 mmol/L). Over the next 2 hours the trend line shifts down slightly and settles in to a new track. Calibration at 6am affirms the sensor and meter are in agreement. Repeated experiments like these, done when the situation allows it, allow the Sugar Surfer to define tiny responses to insulin under normal circumstances. This set of "baseline" experiences will be called upon when circumstances are not routine or normal. It provides the Surfer with a better way to estimate insulin needs and minimize the chances of under or over treating an out of range BG level or trending BG dot line.

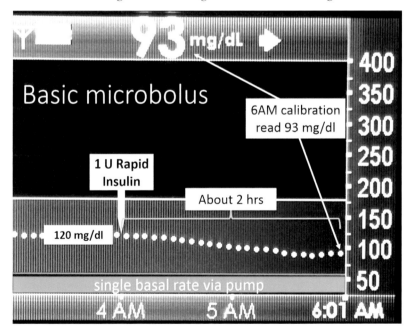

Once you know how sensitive your system is to insulin and carbs, you are prepared to attempt to "steer" the BG trend line. To be safe, you

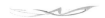

will want to choose a BG target or range that's easy to hit.

I set personal blood sugar targets to "steer" my BG trend line which I call 'pivot points'. An experienced ocean surfer always knows where the beach is no matter what direction board and body are traveling. That same surfer knows the breaking pattern of the wave being ridden. The surfer steers and pivots along the wave crest while maintaining balance on the board. It's not usually a straight line path, but that's not the point.

When I got my first CGM device, the BG target I steered towards was a value of 150 mg/dL (8.3 mmol/L). I would rather err on the high side of a higher target as I learned this new technology. As time moved forward and my Sugar Surfing skills got better, I set lower targets or pivot points to aim at. Today I usually see 100 to 120 mg/dL (5.6 – 11.1 mmol/L) as my ideal pivot point range when at home or work. If I'm working outdoors or doing something involving physical activity, I choose a higher pivot point, at least until the situation changes. Much like the tide is constantly changing, so do my pivot points. The ability to pivot is based on all the other pieces I've discussed so far: proper calibration technique, understanding insulin timing and action, understanding food's effect on my BG, and having a good understanding of basal insulin therapy as well as having somewhat predictable basal action.

Pivot points are not the same thing as your alert settings. Both can and probably should change based on the situation you find yourself. However, these are two very different concepts so be careful not to confuse them.

"Turning a trend" is another way I like to describe glycemic pivoting. It requires frequent CGM screen glances, verifying with a BG check, and understanding the idea of micro-dosing (with insulin) and micro-carbing with fast acting carbohydrates like glucose tablets.

Pivoting is based on the idea that we all live active, often unpredictable lives and we must learn to react just as well (if not better)

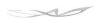

as we pro-act (prepare or act in anticipation of something happening). Blood sugar needs of the body are prone to shift up and down daily for many different reasons, some which can be expected or predicted and others which can't. In both cases, you have no other choice than to react in as timely a fashion possible.

There is no point in trying to know them all, but you should be aware of the biggies:

- food (under or over-estimating what was really eaten)

- food (converting into sugar faster or slower or having a continued effect on BG longer than expected)

- exercise (unexpected or planned)

- insulin (when it's peaking; when it's fading)

- stress (sometimes without realizing it)

Even when you think all of these factors have been accounted for somehow the unpredictable still happens. Here again is the magic of Sugar Surfing combined with frequent glances of your CGM and your willingness to "manage in the moment".

Pivoting forms the "fine tuning" of Sugar Surfing as it relates to maintaining the ability to keep BG trends contained inside a situationally appropriate range that YOU choose and not one that you were given. Just make sure you opt for an easy target range to aim at first. Otherwise you set yourself (or your loved one with diabetes) up for frustration or worse.

Here are several examples of pivoting.

By definition, a pivot is a turn. A basic example follows:

As shown on the illustration on the next page, once I crossed my upper alert threshold of 140 mg/dL (7.8 mmol/L) with a slow upward trend, I took a dose of 4 units of rapid acting insulin. I practice dosing

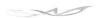

from my upper and lower thresholds this way. They provide a reference point I can better rely on to get a more consistent result. I start with a static BG correction calculation, then modify it based on the situation (rate of rise).

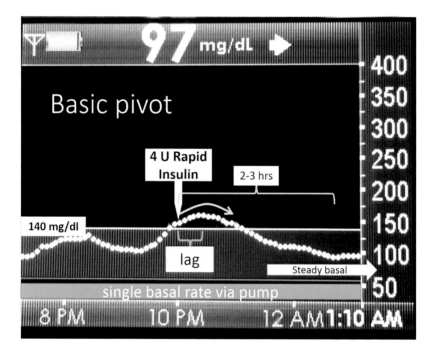

Through repeated practice, I've found 4 units, under normal circumstances, will pivot me back towards my central pivot point of 100 mg/dL (5.6 mmol/L).

However, I find that this is true only when I'm not changing rapidly (the arrow is usually straight across or only angled up, not straight up).

Since my basal rate is not excessive, once my correction insulin has done its work, it deposits me in a pleasant range.

Also notice the lag time between when my dose is taken and any change in blood is noticeable. Correction time for this pivot was about 2 hours.

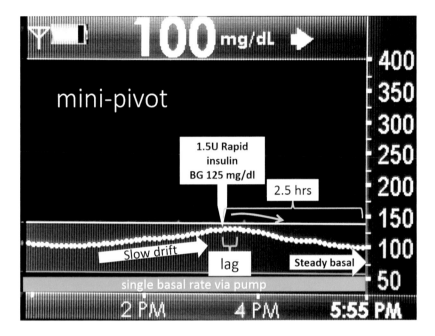

This example forms the basis of what I call a 'mini-pivot'. I used a smaller pivoting dose (1.5 U insulin aspart) and actually dosed myself at 125 mg/dL (6.9 mmol/L) and drifting. As with the previous example, it took two to three hours to correct. My basal rate was properly set. You can see why the basal rate is so important in these examples. Too much basal and there is a constant tendency to drift downward. Too little insulin and the opposite occurs. Minor drifts in both directions are just part of life, with or without diabetes. Without a source of internal insulin, Sugar Surfers must take charge. They practice pivoting, demonstrate patience and learn from mistakes.

As an aside, when would anyone ever dream of taking a dose of rapid acting insulin for a 125 mg/dL (6.9 mmol/L) blood sugar level in the pre-CGM era? I would never have suggested that or done it myself. And I still won't unless it is in a well-trained Sugar Surfer. Glucose sensing changes many of the 'rules' of diabetes management.

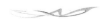

Pivoting is the offspring of micro-bolusing. You can't do one without a working understanding of the other.

Through the use of smaller amounts of insulin (micro-bolusing) or carbs (micro-carbing with fast acting carbs), the trend line can be "steered" around a central "pivot" point. Pivoting takes time and practice to master. But to be an accomplished pivot pro, you need to understand micro-dosing. But first, let's dive into a little more on carbs and pivoting.

Mini-carb pivoting

Recall in Chapter 7 that I asked you to learn micro-carbing as a skill while on a steady or near straight line BG trend line. You might think "What do I do if my BG is trending down and I choose to micro-carb? What then?" That's when you would adjust the amount upwards to offset the rate of fall of the trend line.

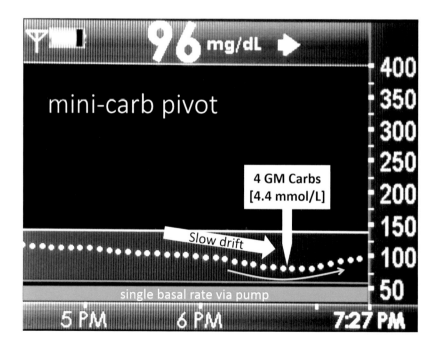

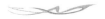

When first trying this on a downward trend line, you can always fall back on the standard teachings of eating 15 grams of fast acting carbs and rechecking in 15 minutes ("The Rule of 15"). It may be too much and you might be overshooting, but it's still better to be safe rather than sorry. Plus, you will remember and make adjustments the next time you are challenged with a similar situation.

Also, experimentations require your extra attention on the way down as well as on the way up. Catching the roller coaster early can give us hours of our day back if only we're willing to sneak a few extra glances at our CGM.

The image on the previous page shows a classic carb pivot. It's a small one, that why I say "mini-pivot". Just 4 grams of carbs (glucose tab) was enough for me. In a younger child the result might be much larger due to a child's smaller size (blood volume).

Carb pivots work faster than insulin due to the quicker action of carbs to raise the sugar level compared to the time it takes for an insulin dose to start to lower it. Practice micro-carbing and carb pivoting when your BG is trending towards your lower alert limit on your sensor. Start at higher levels to begin with to get a feel for how much a small amount of carbs will raise you.

If you are curious, start with eating a standard treatment dose of 15 grams of fast acting carbs while trending straight between 80-120 mg/dL (4.4 - 6.7 mmol/L) and see just how high you go and monitor to see if you stay there for long.

Micro-Bolusing Insulin

Start with a steady BG trend line in the upper half of your target range. There should have been no recent insulin doses for food or correction, just the basal insulin doing its thing. If these conditions are met, then consider taking a very small dose of insulin as a single bolus. "How small?" It totally depends on the person. I started with 1 unit but I could have done less. In my younger patients, the starting point may

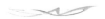

be as little as a tenth of a unit. I like to say "aim small, miss small". After the dose, I wait and watch to see what effect it has over the next two to three hours. Like micro-carbing, I'm not doing anything unusual in regards to activity and I'm not eating either. It took me months to micro-bolus but it was time well spent. I always watched my trend line to observe the effect and repeated the process whenever the situation allowed. I also had more than ample carbs on hand if I trended too low, which by the way, almost never happened.

Many reading this section will be nervous.

"Eating carbs will just raise my BG and that happens more than it should anyway". Our bodies need food to live so let's not fear it. It's way better to understand it and learn how to use it as a tool in our fight against diabetes.

"But I've been told to never take fast acting insulin in any amount except at mealtime or for high BG corrections". Some of you have also been ordered to never take insulin for BG corrections except at meal time only and never inbetween. This is what makes Sugar Surfing a hard concept to some people and it will take some time for most doctors to get comfortable with it.

What I describe next is not an entry level skill. It's always safer for doctors and nurses to say "no" to everyone at least at first and perhaps teach the few exceptions to the rule. What's ironic is that a normally functioning human body produces and releases waves of insulin between meals. The current versions of the artificial pancreas are designed to infuse insulin between meals in response to trending high BG levels just as I'm describing here. The only difference is that a machine will be making the decisions as to how much insulin to give. So why should we not have the opportunity to be trained how to do this properly using the human brain? As I see it, Sugar Surfing is the first step into that new world. But always remember that Sugar Surfing is best done with the help of a well calibrated CGM combined with frequent BG checks with a meter and a motivated and invested patient

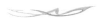

and care team (family).

Please review these examples of micro-correcting or pivoting. Pictures speak volumes. But like micro-carbing, this is a practicable skill. Just do it with full awareness and preparation.

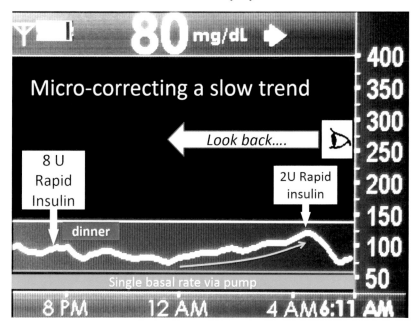

In the example above, I looked back upon waking up and noticed a slow trend that started after I went to sleep. The uptick started after midnight. It was due to a lower carb meal. Also note what a longer time perspective allows you to see... the middle of the night upward curl of the BG trend line. Dinner the night before had been veal parmesan, rice and green beans. Carb ratio was 1 unit of insulin for every 5 grams of carb. Morning meter calibration was spot on. My correction factor at this range is roughly 1:20 (insulin glulisine). Also note that BG trended up from 80 mg/dL to 120 mg/dL (4.4 – 6.7 mmol/L), a 40 point mg/dL difference over 3 hours. This was too slow to change the arrow or to trigger a rise alert but it was a rise nonetheless. I decided to take 2 units of insulin glulisine. About 90 minutes later the trend was turned

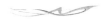

(pivoted) and leveled out on its own at 6 am without the need to micro-carb.

Once you develop a level of comfort with dosing small amounts of carbs and insulin, you are ready to pivot. Like most elements of Sugar Surfing, pivoting is part reactive, part proactive. As a steady trend in the BG is observed that is at least 20 - 30 minutes long, and as the trend line moves away from the central target (pivot point), then a decision is made about whether or not to treat.

The width of the target zone will influence what happens next. My low-high alert range is now set between 60-140 mg/dL (3.3 – 7.8 mmol/L) and 100 mg/dL (5.6 mmol/L) is typically my pivot point.

If I start trending above 120 mg/dL (6.7 mmol/L) towards 140 mg/dL (7.8 mmol/L), I will consider taking some form of action to turn the trend. If the meter BG affirms this rise, I micro-bolus and wait.

If dropping below 80 mg/dL (4.4 mmol/L) I will micro-carb and glance at the response over time.

Using a BG check to confirm the reading, a micro-carb is applied, then time is allowed to pass as the trend line is watched over the next hour or two. Rechecking BG with a meter confirms what is seen on the screen and can be used for additional sensor calibrations as needed.

PROACTIVE-REACTIVE

This slide on the next page sums up many principles of Sugar Surfing. From left to right:

After eating 3 pieces of fried chicken, I reduced my basal insulin delivery rate (a.k.a. "engine brake") to offset a trending low (not shown on the left). I did not take a combo bolus, intentionally. (PROACTIVE MOVE)

Fried chicken tends to create a slow rise for me through the night.

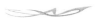

Notice that my high alert threshold is set at 140 mg/dL (7.8 mmol/L) and low alert is 60 mg/dL (3.3 mmol/L). Through careful trial and error, I've gotten comfortable taking 3 units as this threshold is crossed. As you can see, 3 units pivoted me down to 116 (6.4 mmol/L) in a little under 2 hours. When you do this, take your time and start small as you try to turn a rising trend (pivot). (PROACTIVE and REACTIVE)

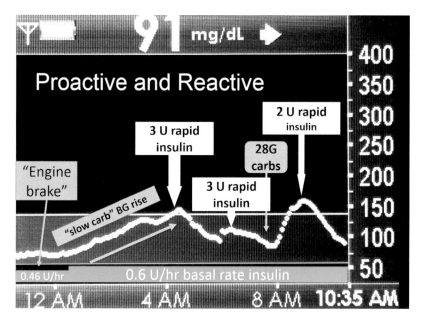

Next, I took my usual 3 unit insulin aspart breakfast dose and "Waited for the Bend"...and waited...and waited. I finally ate my breakfast (28 grams carbs) 90 minutes after my usual 3U dose. Notice the uncharacteristic rise from the meal, which I then addressed with a 2 unit correction at 8:50am. In about 90 minutes the BG gets back to a desirable target zone. (PROACTIVE and REACTIVE)

Here is my main point: notice the variable blood sugar lowering result of 3 units of aspart taken only a couple of hours apart. If I were to only rely on fixed ratios to calculate an insulin dose, imagine how much more unpredictable my glucose control might be. The simple truth is

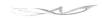

that there is minimal predictability in diabetes control. It's not just the insulin of course, but how my body responds to it. And that can change quite suddenly as you can see here. This is a great example of how I "manage in the moment".

Remember those 3 virtues of Sugar Surfing: Patience, consistency and resilience? These are your surf buddies.

Surf in guilt free waters

By now you've read about the many ways you can purposefully steer a BG trend line, plus safely recover from flux and drift that might have gotten away from you due to a short lapse of attention. Remember, Sugar Surfing is best performed with a guilt free mindset. You put yourself out there and do the best you can. Assigning shame or blame does not make you a better surfer, it only slows down your ability to improve your skills. Even if you miss a few rising or dropping sugar waves and have to paddle back into your target zone, in the end you will still have better overall control of your diabetes than if you weren't surfing at all and playing the static management game.

The rest of this chapter discusses what I consider advanced Sugar Surfing 'moves'. The basic elements of the moves I will describe are partly based on material covered in earlier chapters. It's the intensity, frequency and applying these skills in combination which make them more complex. To me, advanced Sugar Surfing also means an advanced level of personal motivation and maintaining your focus over a longer period of time. Things that require a significant effort or frequency of effort, even though they might be easy to do, must be considered advanced.

Always keep in mind that Sugar Surfing is a process, not a result. The ability to keep the trend line in a range of your choosing depends on how much time and attention you can apply to it all. While this may sound like all you do is hover over your CGM readout, it doesn't have to take that much time. Recall from Chapter 7 that the action of collecting visual information from the CGM is what I call "glancing".

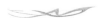

These quick looks can be done virtually anywhere: in bed, while exercising, watching television, in the car, at the movies, or in a meeting. I've counted the number of times I glance. It tends to average 40 - 50 times a day. This is more than the average CGM user I've been told: about 15 - 20 looks a day. But it's the timing of the look and what's done with the information seen on the screen that has the most effect on blood sugar control, not just how many times the screen is viewed. In some ways, this is no different than checking BG with your meter. It's all about what you do with the information you get.

How to glance properly

Each time the CGM screen is viewed, a quick decision is being made. Usually, it's whether to dig deeper for more information. This could mean looking at the dot line along longer or shorter time windows (zooming in and out) to get a proper feel for the overall trend (if any) and how long it's been going on. It might suggest the need to check a BG level with a meter in preparation to act on a rising or dropping BG trend. But as these actions with the sensor are going on, the Surfer is also thinking about the situation at hand. Perhaps it includes the last meal or snack, current or recent physical activities, stress, when the last insulin dose was taken (or how much). It also includes what is expected to happen next: such as the next meal or activity. And this list is far from complete.

My checklist goes like this:

How do I feel?

What am I doing?

What actions will I be doing next?

When did I last eat?

When was my last insulin dose?

Do I need to check a BG?

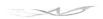

Do I need to micro-carb or micro-bolus insulin?

Where are my carbs? Where is my insulin?

Professional athletes refer to this situational awareness as "having your head in the game". It's an essential part of Sugar Surfing. Not surprisingly, like a muscle, this skill improves and strengthens with time and repetition. It just takes practice and a realization that a screen glance is as much a diabetes self-management skill as injecting a dose of insulin, lancing your finger, or measuring a serving of food.

A screen glance combined with situational awareness results in an action or actions performed by the Surfer. This is the most basic element of Sugar Surfing: the action loop. Actions taken can range from nothing (e.g., "I will wait for more information and glance again in a few minutes") to major changes (e.g., BG check immediately, then choosing and taking a corrective insulin dose followed by more frequent screen glances and meter checks). Just remember, choosing NOT to take action is itself an action. If you think an act of omission is not important, imagine what would happen if you took a dose of mealtime insulin and DIDN'T eat. Or if you ate and DIDN'T take an insulin dose for the meal. See my point?

Action loops

Becoming a competent Sugar Surfer starts with practicing the action loop. If the CGM screen is glanced at 15 times a day, this means there are at least 15 opportunities to act, right? The simple answer is no. That's because Sugar Surfing involves more than only checking a CGM readout. Experienced Surfers are usually in tune with their own behavior patterns, and often recall previous experiences where blood sugar levels went well or didn't. These memories and experiences are perfectly valid Surfing tools by themselves. For example, I carry in my immediate memory when I took my last insulin dose, the type and amount of food I ate (or didn't), and what usual or unusual activities I might be doing (or did). It also might be curiosity that prompts me to glance at my CGM screen more so than any feeling I might have to see

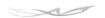

if my BG dot line trend is rising or falling. The sense of seeing my BG in a desirable range and trending in a steady direction makes it attractive to keep doing this. It's self-reinforcing.

The action loop is the engine of Sugar Surfing; like surfing rail to rail. This engine drives the selection and use of a wide range of tools and methods by each Surfer and these are explained throughout this book. These tools are intended to safely steer the BG trend through the day and night. Surfing moves can be performed as few as once a day, but don't expect diabetes control to be that great if you do. The more you keep your head in the game, stay engaged and pace yourself, the better you're able to manipulate your diabetes for the better.

Use your sensor as a biofeedback tool

Over the years I've worn a CGM, I constantly challenge myself to guess which direction my BG trend line is moving before glancing at the screen: up, down or fairly level. At first I was fairly accurate when my BG was clearly falling or rising. But over time, and with lots of practice, I was able to sense the smallest of shifts in my trend line with nearly 100% accuracy. The amazing thing is that I learned to sense minor shifting in my trend line when my BG was not in an extreme range. For example, I can routinely sense a slight downward drift in my BG from 120 to 110 mg/dL (6.7 – 6.1 mmol/L). I can also sense a gradual rise from 90 to 100 mg/dL (5.0 – 5.6 mmol/L). Make note that these abilities are present at BG levels that are not in the low BG (hypoglycemic) range or the high BG (hyperglycemic) range. I practice this every day. Guessing my BG trend direction is a personal challenge I engage in all the time. Like one of Pavlov's dogs, when I reach down to press the button on my CGM I'm making a guess in my mind. And I never get tired of doing it either. I've been witnessed doing a "fist pump" every now and then. It's the little things that empower me since I can experience successes like these throughout the day. After all, it's said that feedback is best delivered when it's immediate. After having type 1 diabetes for almost 50 years, being able to develop and practice this ability is one reason why I am enamored with CGM as a much

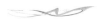

under appreciated biofeedback tool.

Sensing shifting sugars

If you're like me and glance often, then you're also likely to see a rising or falling BG trend before you get too far off track. Many experienced Surfers can even "sense" subtle shifts only to verify by checking the sensor screen and by checking a BG level with the meter.

After almost 50 years with type 1 diabetes I thought I could no longer sense lows. My CGM proved me wrong, but not at first. After wearing my device a few months I developed an intense curiosity of what my BG was doing all the time. I checked the readout dozens of times a day. But I soon turned this into a personal challenge to "guess" the direction of my dot trend line each time before I glanced at it.

The image below shows that as the BG trend is drifting down, areas of the brain can sense this shift. They are not expressed like what you are used to feeling with a low BG (shakes, sweats, rapid pulse) but rather in very subtle changes in mood or attitude in my inner thoughts. I know it sounds strange, but it works. What I've discovered by researching this further is that certain areas of the brain and central nervous system can respond to changing or shifting BG levels that are not just in the areas we define as low or high.

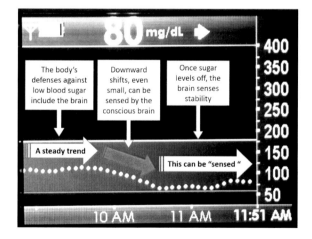

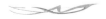

This was one of the greatest, and least developed or understood, benefits of wearing a CGM. Now, when I don't have my CGM on, I can use these inner cues to prompt me to check my BG. As I am now many years into wearing these devices, my abilities have gotten even better. At first, you will notice drops and then verify with a glance and meter check. With time and practice, you may start to feel slow drifts too. Likewise, rapid rises may trigger some inner alerts, even when the BG is under 200 mg/dL (11.1 mmol/L) and going up quickly. Later on, slow rises might catch your attention. The sense of stability or a level trend, is the hardest to sort out. For example, if I'm trending at 80 mg/dL or 150 mg/dL (4.4 or 8.3 mmol/L) and going straight I may have a harder time telling the two apart, but since I'm not dropping or spiking, that's good.

To develop this skill you need time and patience. It took me a year or so to not only discover this was a benefit, but to develop it as another tool in my diabetes arsenal. You can do it faster than I did now that you know this skill can be developed. Using the CGM as a biofeedback tool is a phenomenal confidence builder.

It is an easy game to play. No one needs to know you are doing this. Just before glancing at the CGM readout, think to yourself ,"Am I trending steady, dropping or rising"? Then look and see if you are right. Remember, look at the dot lines, not just the direction arrows. They will not have the sensitivity unless you are changing rapidly in one direction or the other. Just do it before every glance. Within days or weeks you will be surprised with what you can do. I can "feel" a slow drift downward of as little as 10 mg/dL (0.6 mmol/L). Seriously.

But if you are busy or mentally preoccupied with something else or just want to have an early warning heads up, then go ahead and change your alert thresholds and rate of rise and fall alerts to tighter, narrower and more sensitive levels to provide you an early warning of trending highs or lows. You can always change them back in seconds for other situations as needed. Sensor alert thresholds should be adjustable by you based on your unique needs or conditions. This is situational

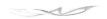

thinking in action and another important Sugar Surfing skill.

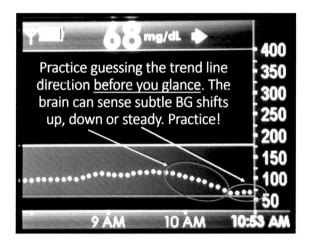

Waiting for the Bend

Once I know how high or low my morning BG level is, plus what I plan to eat, I dose my insulin and "wait for the bend". I show several examples here along with their results. You must have the opportunity to wait and have ready access to your meal, too.

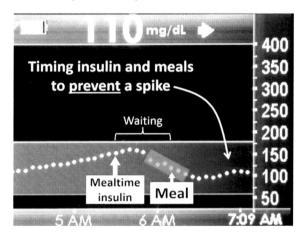

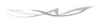

The bend can start anywhere from 15 minutes onward. Sometimes it might not happen at all. Stress, damaged insulin and pump problems are possible culprits.

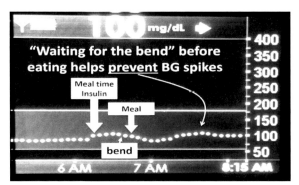

Waiting might not always be possible and sometimes eating must occur with (or even before) any mealtime insulin dose is taken. Just be prepared to manage a later rise or BG spike. I do this as often as I can. It pays off big when I do. However, there are some situations and reasons for not waiting to eat after an insulin dose. I will discuss these below.

First, you must have a well calibrated sensor as already discussed. Second, you must have a source of rapid-acting carbohydrate with you in case your meal somehow fails to materialize on time (to prevent a low). Third, you need to know what you are going to eat plus an estimate of the carbs in the meal to figure out your insulin dose. Fourth, through prior experience you should know how slowly or fast the meal you are about to eat might affect your blood sugar levels (fast, medium or slow). Lastly, you should glance at the sensor trend line often through the meal and afterwards. I may glance at my sensor several times over the span of my meal to monitor my progress and make additional in the moment decisions about taking additional insulin or eating more (or less) food.

When I wait for the bend, I'm trying to neutralize two moving targets which generally want to move in opposite directions: insulin (a BG lowering force) and food (a BG raising force). The goal is to balance

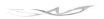

out the sugar raising effect of the meal with the sugar lowering effect of the insulin. "Mission Impossible", you say? It may seem that way at first, but with time and practice and some smart experimenting, you'll be surprised how well you can do it with the help of your own wits, a BG meter and a well-calibrated CGM.

In some ways I've developed a partnership with my sensor. I need to maintain it properly to get the most use from it. I know that the first few days after insertion of a new sensor the blood sugar information can be highly erratic. Remember: Don't stress, assess! I just check BG more often and use that information to teach the sensor with additional smart calibrations as explained in the previous chapter called Waxing Your Board. I don't overdo it either. I know the limitations of my sensor. As a result of my approach to using CGM, I regularly maintain my sensor readings within plus or minus 20 mg/dL (1.1 mmol/L) of my meter readings around 80-85% of the time.

Pre-empting

A basic principle of Sugar Surfing is anticipatory management: thinking and acting to prevent problems. That means remembering past management successes and failures to improve subsequent attempts. It's a constant improvement cycle. The embodiment of this principle is found in pre-empting. As a rising BG trend is occurring, it makes sense to decide if an intervention is needed to keep the trend from getting out of control. Pre-empting applies to using any force known to change BG level or trend direction based on careful analysis of the situation "in the moment". Eating carbs to manage a falling BG trend is a form of pre-empting. Exercising to prevent a trending high from going even higher is another example. But using insulin after a dose has already been given takes us back to the earlier discussions about insulin stacking and even the use of I-chains.

I use another example of a slow acting protein, carb and fat containing meal. This food's effect on my blood sugar was outlasting the insulin dose I had taken earlier.

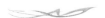

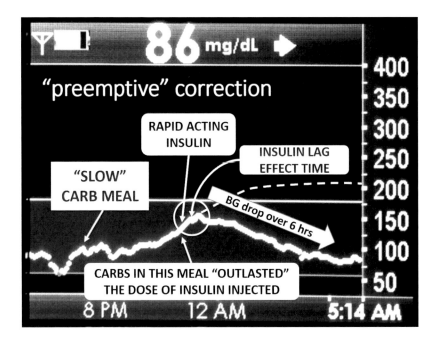

I was also not using an insulin pump in this example. The basal insulin was glargine (Lantus). Selecting from a range of insulin doses that I can use in the range I was in as the BG was trending upward, I took a dose as the BG was on the rise. "Calculated risk"? Yes. Experience had taught me that if I did not act, my BG would be well over 200 mg/dL (11.1 mmol/L) by morning. So I took the preemptive dose and you can see the results that followed. I watched the effect overnight and my alarms typically waken me or my wife. Frankly, I slept well through the night. I had rehearsed situations like this during the day and felt confident I would not have a problem I couldn't deal with. I would not have felt this way at first. This reflects the confidence that comes with Sugar Surfing: an inner sense of control over your diabetes. Respect. Not fear.

Sugar Surfers are constantly learning. The more you know or learn from a previous attempt, the better your next attempt becomes. You might say this is a champion's attitude and I would not argue. Failure is our best teacher. We just have to listen to what it tells us and change.

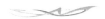

Special tactics

Sugar Surfing uses many tools and strategies to steer the BG levels in the body. The following are some special tools that may help you someday.

Sleep bolus. This deserves another mention. It is discussed in the previous chapter. It's a great way to correct a high BG at night with less risk of middle of the night low blood sugar. The method is elegant and only applies to persons using a functioning insulin pump. To apply a sleep bolus calculate the amount of insulin needed to correct the out of range BG back to target. Then program that amount of correction insulin to be delivered as a square wave or extended bolus over 5 or 6 hours. The correction is more gradual, but the risk of middle of the night low BG is less. To be even more conservative, just take 50% of the insulin you would normally use to correct in that situation. In the morning see how it worked out for you. If your BG stayed too high then next time try 75% and so on.

Engine braking. This is not a surfing term, but it best describes this move. As a slowly drifting low BG looms ahead, an insulin pump basal rate can be temporarily reduced or stopped altogether. Here is an example of an engine brake:

If this action is applied about one hour before a slowly evolving low is happening or during a time when a prior insulin bolus was given, you can possibly prevent the low or at least reduce the severity of the low and make it easier to treat.

Engine brakes require planning and an awareness of what your BG trend line is doing. They are fun to use and can help you avoid having to eat to treat a low. The need for them might be some lingering insulin action from a prior dose, late effect of exercise or just more physical activity in general during the day.

Applying the brakes is usually only needed at most for one to two hours. The amount to reduce the basal rate requires practice.

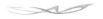

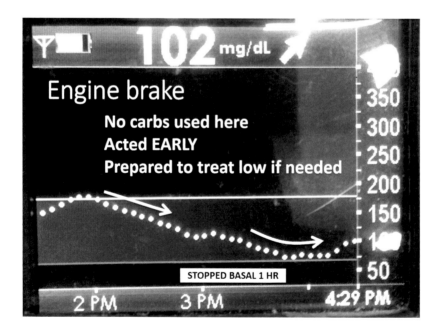

Depending on how fast BG is falling, you might just stop the basal delivery altogether. In the next engine brake example, the BG is dropping but the brake is applied fully (basal rate was suspended entirely for one hour) at a BG of 125 mg/dL (6.9 mmol/L) as a drop from 180 mg/dL (10.0 mmol/L) was occurring. Without carbohydrates, the BG drop slowed down and shifted back up.

Applying an engine brake alone when BG has already crossed into the hypoglycemic range is too late. While helpful, the recommended action would be to treat with fast carbs to raise BG. Just don't over treat and make sure to restart your basal rate once you see the BG improving. If you don't turn the basal rate back on, you are at risk for very high sugar levels and even diabetic ketoacidosis. Never go too long without basal insulin.

The engine brake is similar to the basal rate suspend feature on some new CGM-enabled insulin pumps. If the CGM measures a BG below a pre-set threshold, the pump will suspend all basal insulin delivery and alarm the user of the situation. Engine braking is simply the manual version of that process, but a total suspend or something in-between would be entirely up to you. Experience combined with careful and frequent CGM glancing is required for this move. Also, insulin pumps are advancing in this area quite rapidly as part of the manufacturer's artificial pancreas programs.

I-chains. No, this is not a new product from Apple. It's a unique way to coordinate the dosing of rapid acting insulin when using multi-dose insulin therapy instead of an insulin pump. It's applied to meals with a larger load of slowly digesting carbohydrates. I use one common Texas example of Tex-Mex food. Certain pastas, fried foods and pizza would also be good candidates for I-chaining.

I –chains is the process of timing rapid-acting insulin doses in such a way as to minimally overlap (stack) their effects while providing a steady insulin effect to help the body properly manage the blood sugar due to a large carb, fat and protein-laden meal. In this example, since I

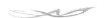

ate a large amount of carbs, I took two doses of mealtime insulin close together at the start. I would not consider this a true insulin stacking since it was done for the same meal.

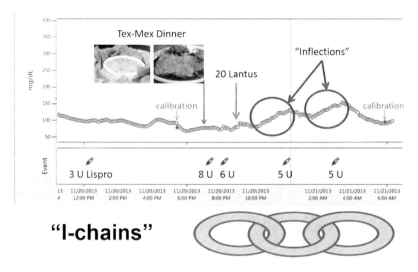

"I-chains"

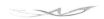

I next closely watched the BG trend line for inflections. As the first trend line was increasing over the course of an hour, I reached my upper alert threshold of 140 mg/dL (7.8 mmol/L). I then took another dose of rapid acting insulin (5 units) and observed the effects over the next two hours. As the BG trend turned upward after two to three hours, I administered another 5 unit dose. My BG meter readings were in range with my sensor readings at each extra dosing point. These two insulin pivots finally brought the trend line back into range by morning.

An I-chain is a manual version of a combination (dual wave) or extended (square wave) bolus from an insulin pump. Careful attention to the CGM trend line is key to its proper use and ultimate success. The estimated duration of insulin action is used to determine the spacing between rapid-acting doses. I've determined by careful observation what the duration of insulin action is for several insulins. Combining that with observed inflection points on the CGM readout suggest if the last dose's "effectiveness" is fading and whether or not a new rapid acting insulin dose should be introduced to keep the pressure on rising blood sugar. I-chains take practice to execute well.

Taking the drop. This is a real ocean surfing term. I apply it to show a more dramatic micro-bolus like effect.

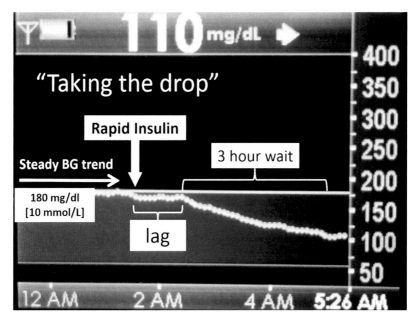

Using my upper range threshold as a starting point, I have rehearsed through repeated trial and error the best average insulin dose that will "drop" me from that point back to a smooth landing in my target zone. I'm aiming at my pivot point in most cases. This example illustrates the concept.

Taking the drop is classically done from a steady baseline as shown here. It's the big brother of the micro-bolus as you are probably thinking. In this example, there was a longer lag time before the drop started. This is not uncommon. The larger the drop, the longer the lag. And it took a full three hours to get back to baseline. As always, this depends on having a well set basal rate. This is illustrated by the level of BG trending before the drop inducing dose of insulin was given.

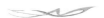

Remember, a basal rate is only meant to maintain stability, NOT drop a BG level on its own. I think many persons with diabetes with chronic low BG problems run a higher basal rate than necessary. This can be an overlooked reason for middle of the night low blood sugars in some people.

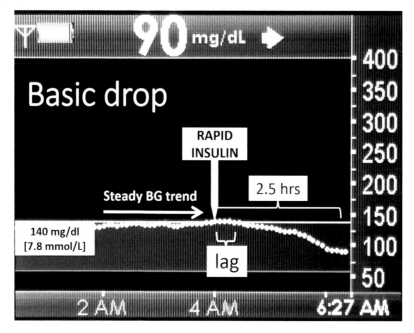

Many of my early drops were practiced from a 180 mg/dL (10 mmol/L) threshold. I eventually moved to a 140 mg/dL (7.8 mmol/L) upper alert limit on my CGM. I've practiced many "dives" from these two starting points. In general, I find 6 units works well for 180 and 3 units for 140. But that is only me. Furthermore, circumstances (food, activity, stress) and general BG trend direction will influence whether I raise or lower these starting doses in each case.

Exercise. One powerful, and at times unpredictable tool to manage type 1 diabetes is exercise. It can be used with many Sugar Surfing moves, like a drop, to lower a BG level with less insulin.

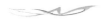

In the examples below, a 4 unit dose is used to drop from a steady trend line on the top image. On the bottom image, half the insulin is used along with the same amount of exercise (walking the dog 4 miles). Using the CGM, the lowering effect can be tracked. Of course always carry fast acting sources of carbs whenever doing any kind of sustained physical activity. Remember that exercise alters estimates for insulin corrections, usually downward, but not always. Through careful trial and error with your CGM you can map your own responses.

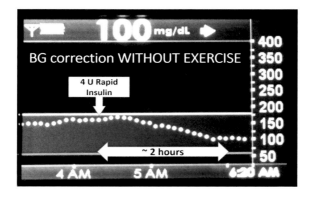

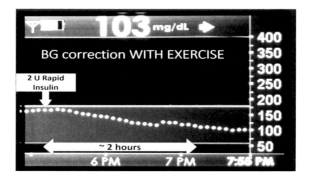

Putting Sugar Surfing to the test.

The following examples are when all my Sugar Surfing skills were put to the test. I annotate each and emphasize key teaching points.

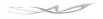

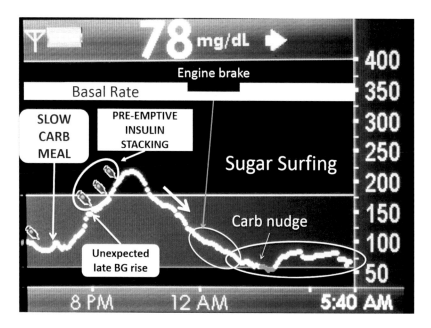

In this example, an unexpected late night rise in my BG (probably due to the sour dough bread), was met with a barrage of preemptive insulin doses (green rectangles) to pivot the rising BG trend and take the drop. Midway down the drop (at 125 mg/dL [6.9 mmol/L]), I tried a small engine brake (40% basal rate reduction for 2 hours) to slow the rate of descent. Nevertheless, a small carb nudge (10 grams of carbs) of grape juice was needed at 2:34 am to bring me back into range where my well set basal rate kept me until morning.

This was a good learning experience. I now engine brake more aggressively with 60 - 100% basal rate reductions.

Each day can be very different

You never dive into the same waters twice. These images done on consecutive days show how variable one day's BG responses can be very different from the next.

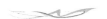

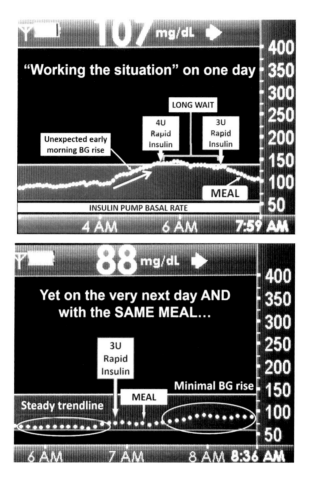

I could speculate many reasons why, but in Sugar Surfing an absolute answer is not always needed to keep moving forward. If I need to take extra insulin, I take it. If I need to wait longer for the bend, I'll wait longer. But sometimes I can't wait and I have to use other Sugar Surfing techniques to correct an unexpected rise or fall in my BG level. My experience is not any different than anyone else. One big time saver for me is that I just don't bother trying to assign blame unless I am certain that an error was made. Then instead of getting upset about it, I fix it and do my best to remember next time. No guilt!

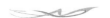

Missed basal insulin dose and recovery

Yes, I missed an insulin dose here. I fell asleep before taking my evening dose of insulin glargine (Lantus). My high alert was set at 180 mg/dL (10 mmol/L) and this is when I discovered my error. Realizing I would soon be awash in high blood sugar and ketones, I took a corrective dose and my scheduled glargine dose (albeit about 5 hours late). And as luck would have it, I experienced a sensor data gap. I checked my BG during that time to make sure I was not overshooting my target. When my sensor came back on line after 2 hours, I was back in my comfort zone. Alert alarms are for more than just picking up lows at night!

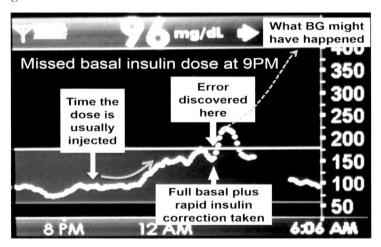

In this example, several missteps contributed to this pattern. First, I should have used a combination bolus with my pump for the meal I ate instead of a large single dose of 17 units of insulin lispro. The larger dose resulted in an effective duration of insulin action of almost 5 hours. Second, I had for some reason set my upper alarm alert too high and forgot to set it back to my usual lower limit. I took a dose that should have caused a reasonable drop and indeed that happened. But it later plateaued in the 170 mg/dL range (9.4 mmol/L). After waiting for an hour to see if a further drop would happen (it didn't), I took another smaller dose which brought me towards my target zone. I also used

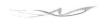

that second dose to cover my breakfast carbs at 7:15 am as a braking maneuver. This also illustrates a two-step drop which is safer in my opinion than a much larger single dose attempt.

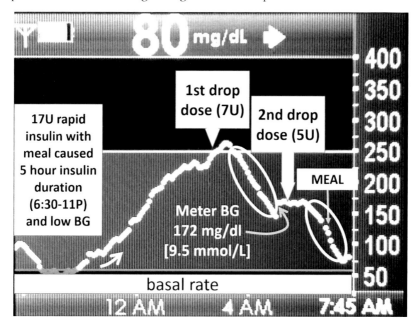

Dining out

I try to keep track of the carbs in my foods but it is not always easy to do. Especially when I eat out and go to special celebrations like a wedding. If I choose to eat at a Mexican wedding buffet or Japanese Hibachi restaurant I'm certain to run into lots of carbohydrates. I could choose to not eat those items of course and go low carb. In these two examples, I ate or ordered what I was craving. I guess you could say I "ate normal". I didn't consume sugary beverages, though.

Most of the time I'm pretty careful about what and how much I eat, but I do love knowing that I can pick and choose those times when I will eat as much as I like without feeling like I'm destined for high blood sugar. My Sugar Surfing skills allows me that ability. I don't abuse it. I'm grateful to have learned and refined these skills.

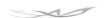

On the screen below, I attended the wedding of a young man I've helped since age 3. At the reception was a Mexican buffet and the wedding cakes of course. I listed what I ate. As my BG started climbing I took a series of 7 small back to back doses (a modified insulin stack), and watched my trend line carefully. I assumed the insulin effect would last at least 5 - 6 hours. I helped things along with another 6 unit rapid acting insulin dose for the wedding cake. Due to the long time it took to contain all those carbs, I took a final nudge to steer my BG back into my zone.

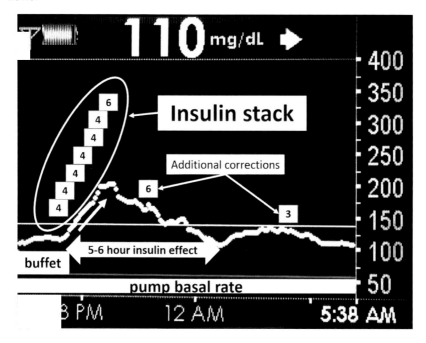

In the example on the next page, I intentionally ate the large stack of fried rice. Based on prior experience I knew fried rice has a strong effect of my blood sugar. I wanted to surf through that wave. Taking a modified insulin stack as the trend was rising, I was able to pivot for a short time before the meal pivoted me back upward. At that time I took 3 more doses over the next few hours to steer me back to home base and my well set basal rate.

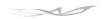

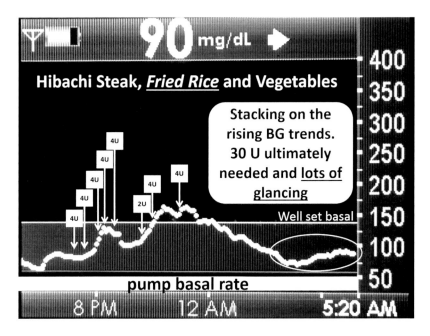

Hibachi Steak, _Fried Rice_ and Vegetables

90 mg/dL ➤

Stacking on the rising BG trends. 30 U ultimately needed and lots of glancing

Well set basal

pump basal rate

In both these examples I was well prepared to deal with low blood sugar. First of all I checked my BG often. Second, I had ample fast acting carbs immediately available to treat a trending low. Third, with my CGM I could see a low coming well before it had a chance to cause me any trouble.

Tired of Surfing, yet? Sometimes it's hard work but worth it!

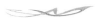

The Future

Chapter 15

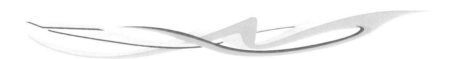

In conclusion, everything you need to become a Pro Surfer is already here so stop waiting for the next cool shiny gadget to change your life. Start today and get on with it.

Having trouble with reimbursement? Be like that dog on a bone. Get your doctor to help you. Find others who have already won the fight and ask them to help you.

Developing your inner surfer combined with daily use of CGM will change your life, today. No more waiting needed. When you do get access to this amazing technology please don't let it sit in a drawer.

Remember, no pump required! Just your commitment and willingness to gain intimate knowledge about your own body through safe experimentation and managing in the moment.

And finally, for crying out loud realize that it's not just a convenient substitute for finger-pricks and a meter. That's what the static method teaches and you've chosen to take a different path... the one toward dynamic diabetes management.

Now consider yourself the newest member of my Surf Colony. You've joined with thousands of others and I'm counting on all of you to not fall back into your old static diabetes management habits. Be dynamic. No guilt! Live a normal life... but be anything but normal.

Surf's Up!

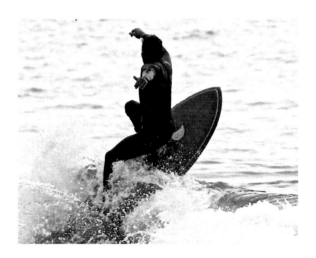

"True happiness is... to enjoy the present, without anxious dependence upon the future."

- Lucius Annaeus Seneca

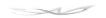

Acknowledgements

Frankly, I never planned to write a book. But when prompted by so many people who read my online diabetes posts to "write a book about all this stuff you call Sugar Surfing", I first thought I would avoid taking it on by asking them to pay for it. So we set up a crowdsourcing campaign and much to my surprise, we quickly raised the capital needed to create this book. As so many of you quickly stepped up with funding for this book, I felt deeply humbled, but then suddenly quite challenged. I wish to acknowledge all those who believed that more people should be able to read all they could about Sugar Surfing, and in one concise place. I'm pleased with this effort and glad that so many people can now get what they asked for.

This book is for everyone living with and caring for anyone with type 1 diabetes. I also wish to dedicate it to my late Mom, Betty Ponder and my Dad Jack Ponder who recently celebrated his 90th joyful birthday, to my wife of almost 30 years Patsy, and to my children Charlotte Ponder, Rachel Hopkins RD, and Jackson Ponder.

I wish to recognize the role that my family played in helping me live well with diabetes. My Mom and Dad, and my younger Sister, Stacey, comprised my first family unit. There is no doubt in my mind that I would not have made it this far in life without their constant love, support and understanding. My wife Patsy and children Charlotte, Rachel and Jackson have enriched my life beyond measure.

I am forever grateful to my professional diabetes mentors Drs. Luther Travis, Ben Brouhard, William J. Daeschner, Jr, William J. "Bill" Riley and Bruce S. Keenan. Dr. Travis led me to the Texas Lions Camp for Children with Diabetes in 1981 which set me on the professional path I travel today. I also never stopped returning to diabetes camp and still serve as Medical Director each summer. Over the years I've met thousands of young people and health care professionals through my affiliation with the Texas Lions Camp. Much of my growth as a diabetes specialist was made possible by my affiliation with this incredible organization.

I also want to acknowledge Barbara J. Schreiner, PhD BC-ADM CDE, Barbara J. Anderson PhD, "The Barbs" as I know them, for all their wisdom and encouragement over the years.

Further, I want to acknowledge Patsy and Bence Reyes, Nelda Caceres, RN CDE and Dr. Peter Kwan for their enduring friendship and loyalty to children with diabetes.

And lastly, I would like to acknowledge my own diabetes. It's been my constant companion since March 1, 1966. This book would have been rather improbable if I didn't have type 1 diabetes. Finally, I try to see each day I've walked the Earth since that date as a gift from God.

Appendix

Terminology

Adhesive. Usually a form of paper or plastic tape with a sticky side that is used to attach an insulin pump catheter, tubeless insulin pump or CGM device to the surface of the body. There are different brands of adhesives on the market. Some persons can develop rashes or skin allergies to some adhesives, called contact dermatitis. This can be a significant problem for wearing any or all of these devices to assist in the management of type 1 diabetes.

Alert alarms. CGM devices can be programmed to notify the user of values crossing or approaching programmed BG thresholds set by the user by using vibratory or auditory alarms with different degrees of sensitivity. Alerts can be set for upper and lower limits that should prompt more attention by the CGM user. Alerts can be easily adjusted by the user as needed to meet whatever situations might arise in the moment.

Alpha cell. The name of the glucagon producing cell(s) located within the Islets of Langerhans in the pancreas.

Apidra (insulin gliusine). A form of rapid acting insulin delivered either by inection or insulin pump.

Basal insulin. Certain types of long-acting and intermediate acting insulin preparations are used to maintain "balance" in blood sugar levels between meals. The action of basal insulin will overlap with meal time insulin but the effect is not usually considered negative. Common basal insulin preparations include insulin glargine (Lantus) and insulin detemir (Levemir). NPH insulin is considered a basal insulin too but tends to have stronger blood sugar lowering effects than the other two.

Basal rate. The delivery of rapid-acting insulin in small amounts every few minutes as programmed through an insulin pump. Basal rates can be changed by programming different settings based on the pump's internal clock. The main purpose of a basal rate is to maintain a steady level of sugar leaving the bloodstream to balance the amount of sugar entering the bloodstream. Even a properly programmed basal rate can be associated with slight up and down shifts in BG trends using a CGM or BG meter. In non-diabetic people, basal insulin changes from day to day.

Beta cell. The name of the insulin-producing cell(s) located within the Islets of Langerhans in the pancreas.

Blood sugar meter. A small, portable device which analyzes a small sample of blood collected from the body and displays the estimated amount of glucose (sugar) in the sample. Readings from meters are not as accurate as laboratory analyzers using blood drawn from a vein. There are dozens of different meters available for use and they may vary in regards to blood sample requirements, time to test, accuracy and precision. The technique used to collect the sample can have a huge effect on the results. This means proper hand washing and collecting a large enough blood sample are very important when using any BG meter.

Bloodstream. The organs and tissues that contain the capillaries, veins and arteries are known as the circulatory system. The liquid that travels within this complex network of vessels is called the bloodstream. The amount of blood in the body will vary based on age, gender, and size. The bloodstream carries oxygen, carbon dioxide, waste products, hormones and thousands of substances that keep the body operating properly. The amount of sugar dissolved into the bloodstream at a given instant is quite small. This is because sugar is constantly entering and leaving the bloodstream.

Bolus. A dose of rapid-acting insulin taken for any reason (meal, snack, or to correct an out of range BG value). A bolus can be taken as an injection or delivered through an insulin pump. Pump boluses can be given all at once (standard bolus) or over a period of time (extended or combination bolus) which is programmed by the pump user and based on the situation. Insulin boluses are given before most meals to get the best results in reducing the rise in sugar levels after a meal. But there are special exceptions to this recommendation.

Calibration. The action of comparing BG information displayed by a CGM device with a standard BG meter reading. In science and technology, measurement devices are occasionally compared to a so-called "gold standard" which represents the most accurate measurement possible. This provides the sensor with a way to match the glucose value in the interstitial fluid to the amount of sugar which is actually present in the blood at the same time. There are many things that can be done well, or done poorly, when it comes to proper CGM calibration. The major challenge of calibrating CGM devices with home BG meters is how carefully the blood sample is collected, how well the meter is used (maintained) and the acceptable error that exists according to the manufacturers design and which has been deemed acceptable by regulatory agencies. See Chapter 6 for more on calibration.

Carbs. Carbohydrates. One of the 3 macronutrients in the human diet. Each gram of carbohydrate contains 4 calories of energy. Carbs are mostly converted to glucose by the body. The speed at which this conversion happens depends on the type of carbohydrate, how it's prepared, what else was eaten with it and even how well it was chewed.

Cell. The smallest unit of life within the body. Each cell contains all the chemical instructions for life in the form of DNA, which is located in a structure called the cell nucleus. Cells are often part of larger tissues called organs which may perform special jobs for the body. They can also be separate and apart, like red or white blood cells. Some cells possess insulin receptors and others to not. For example, red blood cells and nerve tissue do not need insulin to take in sugar for energy or growth.

CGM. Continuous Glucose Monitor. This is a device system which samples the amount of glucose (sugar) in the tissues underneath the skin, not the bloodstream. The area being measured is called the interstitial fluid. Sugar levels in the interstitial fluid are usually in balance with the levels of sugar in the blood. But changes in blood sugar levels up or down will be reflected with a lag as read by the CGM. This time delay can is generally 12-15 minutes behind intravenous blood sugar levels. A CGM uses a sensing device placed into the interstitial space, usually by the user. A reusable transmitter is attached to the sensor (a wire filament designed to couple with the transmitter - the sensor portion is disposable). The transmitter sends a radio signal to a receiving device (either a separate device or incorporated into an insulin pump) which then displays the estimate of the glucose reading on a screen in the form of a number, direction of change arrow, rate of change indicator and a series of points along a graph with time along the bottom and the range of sugar readings on the left. It is increasingly being used in combination with an insulin pump to suspend the pump's insulin delivery when low blood sugar is either measured or predicted. The CGM is a major component of 'artificial pancreas' research.

Correction bolus. A dose of rapid-acting insulin taken by injection or through an insulin pump, intended to lower or "correct" an out of target BG level discovered by careful CGM glancing and BG checking with a meter. Correction boluses require time to take full effect, usually 2-3 hours, and should be carefully monitored using the CGM and verified as needed by BG checking with a meter. Correction boluses can only be used with a rapid (lispro, aspart or glulisine) or fast acting insulin (Regular insulin).

Correction Factor (CF). A mathematical ratio that is assigned to a patient by the diabetes doctor. It's expressed as "take 1 unit of rapid-acting insulin for every BG increment "Y' (in mg/dL or mmol/L) above a 'target' BG value of 'Z' (in mg/dL or mmol/L)". There are formulas used to estimate this value, but many of these are assigned by doctors based simply on personal experience or other non-mathematical means. This is a 'static formula' and how well it works (or doesn't) is affected by several factors including; a) the patient's ability to properly measure a BG level and b) the level of independence given to the patient or family to take insulin between meals. There are ways to verify the effectiveness of the correction factor but these are rarely used in practice. Sugar Surfing incorporates the notion of a correction factor only a starting point or generalized suggestion.

Counter-regulatory. Any hormone or body system which acts to oppose the action of insulin's lowering effect on blood sugar levels. Insulin is the major force that lowers blood sugar by helping move sugar out of the bloodstream and into the cells. It also acts on body organs that actually create or release sugar (such as the liver, muscles and kidneys) to block them from releasing sugar into the bloodstream. The hormone forces which oppose the action of insulin (i.e., act to raise sugar levels in the blood) include glucagon, adrenaline, growth hormone and cortisol, to name only a few. Collectively, these hormones are called 'counter-regulatory' since their actions serve to oppose or "counter" the effect of insulin's lowering effect on sugar. In a person without diabetes, blood sugars are in a constant ebb and flow as a result of the back and forth actions of insulin and counter-regulatory hormones on blood sugar levels.

DCCT. Diabetes Control and Complications Trial. A US based national study begun in the 1980's which answered the question whether improved diabetes control was associated with a lower risk of developing long term diabetes complications or slower progression of existing complications (of the eyes, nerves or kidneys). The results showed that maintaining a lower A1C value over time slows the rate of development or progression of diabetes complications. However, lower A1C levels were generally associated with a greater risk of significant low blood sugar events happening (hypoglycemia).

Diabetes. The word as used throughout this book refers to type 1 diabetes.

Diabetes mellitus. A condition that is caused by the inability of the body to properly manage sugar levels. There are many different ways diabetes can happen. The two most common types of diabetes are called type 1 diabetes (formerly called juvenile-onset or insulin-dependent) and type 2 diabetes (formerly called adult-onset or non-insulin dependent). Diabetes mellitus in one form or another will affect one in four people in their lifetime.

Drift. A Sugar Surfing term. Intended to reflect a gradual rise or fall in blood sugar levels. Drift can occur at any time of the day and is gradual in its appearance. Drift is best revealed by careful glances of the CGM readout. Drift can happen over many hours.

Duration of insulin action (DIA). A method of assigning a numerical value to a dose of fast or rapid-acting insulin that can be used to determine how quickly a dose of that insulin will lose its ability to lower blood sugar levels. Also known as 'insulin on board' or 'bolus on board'. The value is expressed in hours. For example, a DIA of 4 hours states that for each hour following a dose of that insulin, one fourth of that insulin's blood sugar lowering effect will be gone. This factor is used by advanced basal-bolus and pump users to lower (pro rate) the amount of insulin needed for an insulin correction dose if the correction is needed while a recent insulin dose is still considered "active". In reality, fast acting insulin types do not have a steady equal effect throughout their DIA. Rather, there is an approximation of a bell curve with a peak at or near the middle of the DIA.

Dynamic diabetes management. (As opposed to static diabetes management). This is a self care methodology based on the assumption that the patient's diabetes care needs shift throughout the day and day-to-day. It views preset insulin ratios and dosing formulas and meal prescriptions simply as starting points for individualized decision making. BG results are often changing or shaping next steps in care. Virtually no new type 1 diabetes patients are instructed dynamic management principles since static care principles are so much easier to teach. Many people never learn to manage dynamically. Sugar Surfing is the full expression of dynamic diabetes management. To my knowledge, I am the first qualified health care professional to identify, formalize and teach this method. My own unique version of it is called, "Sugar Surfing".

Engine braking. A Sugar Surfing term. As a slow downward drifting BG trend is seen on a CGM readout, a short term (1 - 2 hour) reduction in the basal rate (using an insulin pump) can be used to slow the rate of fall without using a carbohydrate snack, or at a minimum require less carbohydrate to treat the impending low. The amount of basal rate reduction can be between 10-100% (100% means Suspend or giving no insulin for some period of time) based on how fast the downward trend is occurring. Engine braking is not useful if the low BG is imminent. It's usually best applied when the BG is 100 mg/dL (5.6mmol/L) or higher, but clearly drifting down.

Fats. One of the 3 macronutrients in the human diet. Each gram of fat contains 9 calories of energy. Fats can be converted to sugar, but only in very, very small amounts. Most fats contain a small fragment that can be converted into sugar by the liver and other tissues. Fat eaten with a meal containing carbs acts to slow down the process of digestion and can delay the rise in blood sugar after the meal.

Flow. As a Sugar Surfing term, this means the general direction and pattern of a BG trend line viewed on a CGM device. These devices remain (at best) close estimates of BG levels in the bloodstream. Sugar Surfers aim to keep the "flow" of their BG tracings within a self-chosen upper and lower range, but understand that sometimes this does not happen. In those cases, Surfing expertise is needed to steer the BG trend line safely back into range. One goal of Sugar Surfing is to learn how to control the flow of one's own BG patterns through a deeper understanding of the forces that drive blood sugar levels up and down.

Flux. A Sugar Surfing term. Intended to reflect a RAPID rise or drop in blood sugar levels. Flux is not necessarily associated with changes in blood sugar with meals and can happen at any time of the day. Flux is best revealed by frequent glances around times when BG changes are more likely to occur, such as after meals and insulin, during physical activity, stress and illness. The more stable and subtle cousin of Flux is Drift.

Getting ahead of the wave. A euphemism for pre-emptive diabetes self care. It's based on careful attention to the CGM trend line combined with a thorough understanding of one's own glycemic patterns and responses to insulin, food, stress, and exercise. Pre-emptive care aims to minimize large drops or spikes in BG patterns by preventing their full expression as the event is occurring. It is a highly proactive Sugar Surfing action.

Glancing. The act of briefly looking at a CGM receiver readout in real time is called glancing. With practice, the user can see the general direction of the trend line, the CGM's estimate of the current sugar level and an arrow displaying the general trend of the line over the last several minutes or data collection cycles. Experienced Sugar Surfers often average many more glances (40 – 50) each day versus the average user of CGM (10 - 20). Glances can quickly become more thoughtful and calculating if an abnormal trend is seen.

Glucagon. This is a hormone made and released from areas of the pancreas called islets. Glucagon is a protein (like insulin). Glucagon released into the blood is taken to cells where it attaches to receptors on the surface of cells. Glucagon has many jobs within the body, but most of them act to raise sugar levels in the blood. In that respect, glucagon has opposite effects of insulin on lowering sugar levels. Glucagon can be given as an injection to treat a low blood sugar due to too much insulin. Glucagon is also at the heart of artificial pancreas research where it is used in a secondary insulin pump as a counter-regulatory agent whereby small doses in the presence of low or predicted low blood sugar causes the liver to release glucose into the blood stream. a hormone given subcutaneously using an insulin syringe causing rapid deployment of the body's stored glycogen reserves. It is used when patients are incoherent or unconscious and not able to ingest rapid acting carbohydrates via the mouth in a safe manner. Another method of use for glucagon is referred to as mini-dose glucagon.

Glucose. One form of chemical energy used by cells. The chemical bonds which make up the glucose molecule have powerful energy that is released when the molecule is broken down inside the cell. Cells can break and make glucose at the same time. Insulin helps many cells take in glucose so that it can be used for energy and growth.

Glycemic index (GI). A method used to describe the speed at which a carbohydrate food is converted to sugar (glucose) after eating. In general, higher GI foods convert to sugar faster. Ratings for individual foods can be found online. Since meals are a combination of foods with different glycemic indexes, the term Glycemic load has been used to better describe the blood sugar raising effect of a meal.

Hemoglobin A1C. This is a measure of the average blood sugar level over the past several months. This is a blood test that can be collected from a vein or a finger stick blood sample. All persons have an A1C level with or without diabetes. Non-diabetic A1C levels are considered under 6.5%. The A1C does not measure the up and down qualities of blood sugar; only an estimate of the average. There are many things that will interfere with the interpretation of the A1C including certain diseases and blood disorders. Research has proven the A1C to be a helpful tool for monitoring the management of diabetes but it is only one of several tools that should be used.

Humalog (insulin lispro). A form of rapid acting insulin delivered either by inection or insulin pump.

Hyperglycemia. High blood sugar. Hyperglycemia is defined several ways. A non-diabetic person should awaken each day after not eating overnight, with a BG value of under 100 mg/dL (5.6 mmol/L). Two hours after completing a meal a non-d person should have a BG under 140 mg/dL (7.8 mmol/L) . Finally, at any time of the day a random BG level should be under 200 mg/dL (11.1   mmol/L). But persons with diabetes will define high BG levels based on age, situation and some adjustment in the non-d levels outlined above. Over time, high blood sugars can result in damage to body organs in adults and poor growth in children. In the short term, high BG causes increased thirst, more frequent urination, and an increased risk of infection. Sugar Surfing aims to reduce hyperglycemia by using CGM trend information to make preemptive choices and actions to blunt or prevent high blood sugar flux and drift.

Hypoglycemia. Low blood sugar. The formal definition of low blood sugar in persons with diabetes depends on age. The biological definition of hypoglycemia is usually lower than what is used in practical diabetes management. Most adults consider BG under 70 mg/dL (3.9 mmol/L) as low, although this is not a medical definition of hypoglycemia in non-diabetic persons. Parents of toddlers with diabetes might consider a BG of 85 mg/dL (4.7 mmol/L) as low, but again this is not true hypoglycemia. The sensation of a falling blood sugar level is not the same thing as hypoglycemia. Most diabetes specialists view hypoglycemia as mild, moderate and severe. Mild low blood sugar is common in most persons with type 1 diabetes. In these cases, the low is sensed, verified by BG meter and self-treated with fast-acting sugar or food. In moderate hypoglycemia the person may recognize the low but might need to intervene before the sugar drops much lower. In some cases the moderately low person might behave differently or may even deny he/she is having trouble. In severe hypoglycemia the person is not really capable of self-treatment and is at risk for loss of consciousness, seizure-like activity, or death (which is very rare).

Hypoglycemic seizures. These occur when blood sugar is too low to maintain normal brain electrical activity. Brain cells do malfunction and misfire when sugar falls too low. Signs of low brain sugar that precede a low sugar seizure include sleepiness, irritability, confusion, slurred speech or twitching movements. Missed or delayed meals or too much insulin are usual causes. Treating severe lows with an injection of glucagon is best done when the person is not able to safely swallow anything by mouth. Don't use a full dose of glucagon in an alert cooperative person with mild hypoglycemia if they can safely drink or chew food.

I-chains. A series of micro-bolus injections over time with the goal of matching the breakdown of food into glucose in the body. This is performed using an insulin syringe and is intended to approximate the extended delivery option. Also, a Sugar Surfing term used to express the concept of duration as it relates to a series of effective rapid-acting insulin actions. By carefully watching inflection points using a CGM device following an insulin bolus, and a slow-acting meal, the duration of effective insulin action can be estimated. This allows the user to consider administering a supplemental insulin dose to prevent a late rise in blood sugar levels due to a meal or food which takes a long time to convert fully into sugar. Therefore, "I-chains" can be overlapped or linked to provide a prolonged duration of insulin action. This would be the functional equivalent of an extended insulin bolus using an insulin pump. I-chains are an advanced Sugar Surfing concept. commonly available (yet seldom used) in insulin pumps.

Inflection point. When looking at a CGM screen, the dots form a line or curve. An inflection point is where there is a turning of the dot curve in a new direction, or inflection, indicating that BG levels are beginning to move or "trend" in a new direction.

Infusion site. The actual location on the body where an insulin pump catheter is placed. Also, the skin and tissue surrounding the catheter itself. Proper function of a pump catheter relies on a snug seal between the catheter and the skin at the infusion site. A common problem with infusion sites is 'tunneling'. See further on.

Insulin pump. A programmable electro-mechanical device that delivers rapid-acting insulin to a person with diabetes through a small catheter (aka cannula) placed under the skin. The catheter site is changed every 2 - 4 days. A pump delivers insulin in a near-continuous fashion (basal rate) and as programmed by the user to provide insulin for meals, snacks and to "correct" out of range blood sugar readings or trends. Some insulin pumps are integrated with CGM devices. High quality insulin pump use requires proper training, start up training, and ongoing support, advanced skills training, motivation and frequent action.

Insulin Resistance. Affects about one in four Americans. It develops early in life and can wax and wane over time based on weight, health status, activity levels, and medications. It can complicate ANY form of diabetes and should be considered a life long challenge. This condition causes the tissues of the body to require more insulin to do the same work as a non-insulin resistant person. Therefore, insulin levels in the blood of non-diabetics are chronically higher. Not all tissues are insulin resistant. Some organs (like the brain) respond to these high insulin levels by increasing the body's weight set point.

Insulin to carb ratio (I:CHO or I:C). A mathematical ratio that is assigned to a patient by the diabetes doctor. It's expressed as "take 'X' units of rapid-acting insulin for 'Y' grams of carbohydrate to be eaten". There are formulas used to estimate this value, but many are assigned by doctors based on personal experience or non-mathematical means. This is a 'static formula' and how well it works (or doesn't) is affected by factors like a) the patient's ability to properly count carbohydrates, b) the timing of the insulin dose compared to when the food is eaten, and c) factors such as the glycemic index or load of the food or meal. There are ways to verify the effectiveness of the I:CHO ratio but these are rarely used in practice. Sugar Surfing builds on the insulin to carb ratio as a starting point, only.

Insulin. Insulin is a hormone made and released from areas of the pancreas called islets. Insulin is a protein and can be damaged by heat or freezing. Insulin in the blood is taken to cells where it attaches to receptors on the surface of cells. This allows sugar to enter cells for energy and growth.

Intermediate insulin. Another name for NPH insulin. This insulin was the first "longer acting" insulin to be created in the 1940's. It is cloudy in appearance. Its onset of action is about 2 - 4 hours and it usually peaks in 10 - 12 hours. Its duration of action is 18 - 24 hours. There used to be another form of intermediate insulin that I used called

Lente, which acted similar to NPH (an acronym for Neutral Protamine Hagedorn). This was actually a breakthrough discovery. Before NPH, the only insulin for injection was fast-acting Regular insulin, which was extracted from the pancreas of cows, pigs or sheep. NPH insulin was used in many ways like insulin glargine and insulin levemir are used today. Unlike glargine and levemir, NPH did have a noticeable peak activity which made it important to stay on schedule with meals. If not, low blood sugar could be the result. NPH is still used today as part of premixed insulins such as 70/30 and 75/25 insulin where it comprises 70% or 75% of a mixture with faster acting insulin preparations. In some countries this percentage is changed (e.g., 50-50 or 60-40). The action of intermediate insulin is variable from day to day, which is one reason it is not as popular today.

Lantus (insulin glargine). A form of basal insulin delivered by injection.

Levemir (insulin detemir). A form of basal insulin delivered by injection.

Liver. A large organ on the right upper side of the belly. Among its many important roles in our wellbeing, a healthy liver plays a role in regulating blood sugar levels between meals, overnight, during exercise, and after long periods of not eating. The liver responds to the effect of both insulin, glucagon and many other hormones, chemicals and nutrients. In the absence of food, the liver raises blood sugar levels. Stress hormones also tell the liver to make and release sugar.

Multiple Dose Insulin (MDI). This is the method of insulin dosing used by most persons with type 1 diabetes. It involves the use of basal insulin to meet the insulin needs of the body (which are constant throughout the day) combined with meal time "bolus" insulin doses. It is designed to help the body properly metabolize the sugar and other energy that comes from eating a meal or large snack.

Mealtime insulin. Rapid-acting insulin (or fast acting) is taken before, during, or after a meal (depending on the circumstances) to assist in the process of managing the rise in blood sugar that can occur after eating food or drink containing nutrients known to raise sugar levels (mostly carbohydrates). The impact of mealtime insulin on BG control is best measured 2 - 3 hours after the dose and meal, combined with either frequent BG meter checks or use of a CGM device.

Micro-carbing. Taking very small amounts of carbohydrate, usually less than 5 grams, of fast acting carbs like candy, sugar or a glucose tablet. For example, on a very steady baseline BG trend, say my CGM sensor reads 62 mg/dL (3.4 mmol/L), I once consumed 2 Pez candies from my trusty Hello Kitty dispenser. Twenty minutes later I was up to 70 mg/dL (3.9 mmol/L). The actual accuracy of these numbers may be debatable but the fact that this act effected my BG direction was unmistakeable. As you can see, more experimentation is needed. The point is that even 1 - 2 gram carb "nudges" do seem to be possible and measurable. The practicality of them remains to be proven.

Mini-dose glucagon. A procedure involving the hormone glucagon given in small age appropriate dosage subcutaneously using an insulin syringe. It is used on rare occasions when patients are having difficulty in sustaining normal blood sugar in avoidance of stubbornly low blood sugar levels but are otherwise not incoherent or unconscious.

Novolog (insulin aspart). A form of rapid acting insulin delivered either by inection or insulin pump.

Nudge. Making small changes in food, activity or insulin to make small changes in the shape and direction of the BG trend line on a CGM device. Nudging is a Sugar Surfing term that more advanced surfers use to manipulate their BG tracings over the course of a day. It is the smaller piece of the larger process of glycemic pivoting. Nudging and pivoting are terms some might consider to have the same meaning.

Pancreas. An organ about the size of the palm of the hand, located in the abdomen behind the stomach. The pancreas produces many important enzymes and dozens of hormones needed for the proper digestion and absorption of food both after and between meals. Most of the substance of the pancreas is dedicated to making and releasing digestive enzymes into the intestine. Only a small amount of the pancreas (1%) produces hormones which travel throughout the bloodstream. Many of these hormones are produced in clusters or balls of cells called the Islets of Langerhans which are scattered throughout the pancreas from its head to tail. There are over one million islets located in a healthy working pancreas.

Pattern management. Periodic review of blood while investigating for recurring similarities at time of day or possibly day of week under similar circumstances and regimen.

Pivoting. A Sugar Surfing term. The action of using insulin, food and activity in varying amounts and duration to turn around a trending BG pattern on a CGM (or frequently measured BG values from a standard meter) is called pivoting. To pivot, the Surfer must have situational awareness of the direction rate of change of the BG trend line. The up or down BG trend is best verified with a BG meter result. A choice is made as to how to influence the direction of the trend (insulin, food, activity) and the Surfer then carefully watches the trend line as it changes (or doesn't) and continues to manage the situation to influence the direction of the trend line as desired. Pivoting on top of a reliable and well set basal profile is the core principle underlying Sugar Surfing.

Preemptive. The act of taking a corrective action in advance or in anticipation of a result. The intent being that the result of that action will change (usually for the better) the outcome in some measurable way. For example, taking a pre-emptive carbohydrate snack as a BG trend line is rapidly falling but not yet into the range of true hypoglycemia or low blood sugar. Conversely, taking a supplemental insulin dose as a BG trend rises upwards past a predetermined threshold would also be considered a preemptive Sugar Surfing move. In both examples, close follow up and BG checks are required for maximum safety.

Protein. One of the 3 macronutrients in the human diet. Each gram of protein contains 4 calories of energy. Protein can be converted to sugar. This process can be seen using a CGM and careful attention to the trend line for hours after eating. As protein is digested, many of its smaller parts are converted into sugar by the liver and other tissues. Protein eaten with a meal containing carbs acts to slow down the process of digestion and can delay the rise in blood sugar after the meal. How well you chew your food has a direct impact on the conversion of protein into sugar.

Pump catheter (aka cannula). A plastic or metal tube inserted under the skin and attached to the skin by adhesive. The catheter is attached to a length of tubing which connects to an insulin pump containing a reservoir of rapid-acting insulin. The catheter might be part of a tubeless pump system which connects directly to the pump and its insulin reservoir. Many pumps allow the pump user to detach the tubing from the catheter for short periods of time for bathing, showering or certain types of physical activity.

Rapid acting insulin. Insulin preparations are described based on how quickly they start to have an effect on the body. Insulin lispro (Humalog), insulin aspart (Novolog) and insulin glulisine (Apidra) are available types of rapid-acting insulin for use by patients with diabetes. These insulins are only to be taken as an injection (or through an insulin pump) and are not to be taken by vein or inhaled. Rapid-acting insulin is able to get into the bloodstream in 5 - 10 minutes, but the blood sugar lowering effects take longer to happen, usually 15 - 20 minutes just to become noticeable. Most rapid-acting insulins work best (peak) 60 - 90 minutes after injected. Their blood sugar lowering effect will also vary based on the amount injected, how they are delivered (e.g., extended and combination boluses through an insulin pump), the starting blood sugar level when injected and how long the body has been at a given blood sugar level (i.e. - extended durations of high blood sugar may desensitize the body to insulin).

Readout. The screen displaying the data collected from a CGM device. The readout can be part of a pump designed to receive the information, on a dedicated receiver device, to an enabled smart phone, a smart phone app, or through wireless devices which can send the data via the internet to a number of enabled receiving devices (phones, tablets, PC's and even fitness tracker bracelets).

Regimen. The sum of all standard operations for any given patient including blood sugar checks, insulin dosing, meal plan and activity.

Shred. A Sugar Surfing term which describes the act of self-managing diabetes with a CGM or frequent BG monitoring in such a way that most (if not all) forces that would result in poor BG control are prevented, managed early, or corrected more effectively and accurately before they can cause trouble. It's another way of taking ownership of one's diabetes with the assistance of a CGM device, proper training, and LOTS of PRACTICE.

Sleep bolus. When a correction dose of insulin is delivered through an insulin pump, it is typically delivered all at once. Sleep bolus is a modification of this process. The dose of insulin calculated to "correct" an out of range BG level is delivered via the pump as an extended or square wave bolus over 5 - 6 hours. This results in a more gradual decline in BG results. It's called a sleep bolus since it was created at a Summer diabetes camp as a method to correct a high BG discovered before bedtime or at midnight. Rather than have a dose of rapid acting insulin peak overnight and risk low blood sugar, an extended period of insulin delivery reduces the risk of such a low while still achieving the intended purpose of normalizing the high BG level. This can be safer than giving the full dose all at once at a time when everyone is sleeping and unavailable to notice or help in the event of a subsequent severe low blood sugar event.

Self Monitoring Blood Glucose (SMBG). The action of checking a blood sugar level by a person trained in the proper use of a commercial blood sugar meter using a sample of blood collected from a capillary in the fingers, arms or legs using a lancet device.

Stacking. Refers to the intentional or accidental overlapping of the blood sugar lowering effects of rapid-acting insulin preparations (lispro, aspart, glulisine). The term's historical meaning is to describe a scenario of overlapping insulin doses which have the effect of increased downward pressure on blood sugar. The risk of stacking is that a patient who is not mindful will experience unexpected low blood sugar or a prolonged blood sugar lowering problem. In reality, insulin levels overlap often, but under most circumstances this is intentional (such as a combination or dual wave insulin bolus) or part of standard diabetes care (basal-bolus insulin therapy).

Static diabetes management. As opposed to dynamic diabetes management. Static diabetes self care is based on the assumption that the patient's diabetes care needs remain fairly constant over time from day to day. It relies primarily on pre-set insulin ratios and dosing formulas and meal prescriptions that are not immediately changed in response to the results they generate. Virtually all type 1 diabetes patients are introduced to static management principles at first. Many never learn to manage dynamically. Sugar Surfing is the full expression of dynamic diabetes management.

Static vs Dynamic Diabetes Management. Static is scripted in advance. Dynamic is more dependent on the situation or circumstances. Static is easier to teach. Dynamic care requires training, insight and ongoing support. Static favors concrete thinking. Dynamic encourages abstract thinking and problem solving. Static can work with minimal motivation. Dynamic improves and grows with ongoing motivation. Static is less time intensive. Dynamic care is more time intensive. In Static care, outcomes don't immediately influence following actions. In Dynamic care results constantly reshape following actions. Static care = conventional diabetes management. Static tends to be "non-empowered care". Dynamic is "empowered care". Dynamic care = SUGAR SURFING.

Sugar Surfing. A trademarked name given by Stephen Ponder to the collection of knowledge, tools, and experience used to practice dynamic diabetes management using data from frequent BG meter checks or preferably a well calibrated CGM device in combination with a calibrated blood sugar meter. Sugar Surfing does not depend on the method of insulin delivery (pump or injection).

Taking the drop. This is an advanced Sugar Surfing term. The drop is usually started from a fairly straight trending BG pattern on a CGM, verified by meter check. It's usually done at a practiced height multiple times to develop proficiency. For example, taking the drop starting from a steady 200 mg/dL (11.1 mmol/L), 180 mg/dL (10.0 mmol/L) or even 140 mg/dL (7.8 mmol/L) straight line trend for at least an hour. Select a starting point that usually matches with the high alert threshold you've programmed on the sensor. Next, a correction dose of insulin is given and the BG trend line watched frequently over the next 2 - 3 hours as the BG trend line falls towards its target and then levels off in the desired range. Taking the drop requires much practice. It starts with selecting a starting point (mentioned above), then using standard correction doses based on what the doctor has prescribed. Through repeated practice, and starting with smaller doses at first, the Surfer builds confidence around a situation that might happen occasionally and which might require a very skilled correction back to target. Through this highly personalized series of drop attempts, Surfers will eventually find their own drop correction doses based on the different starting point of the steady elevated BG trend.

Teamwork. Family unity, adopting a nonjudgmental attitude, open communication, and task sharing are common traits of this situation. I've consistently seen this displayed by families of well managed kids and teens. As a team, we aim to help persons shed as much guilt, anger, and fear about their diabetes as they can release, as soon as they can. These darker emotions act as a cancer on the ability of families to travel the path to mastering diabetes in themselves and in helping their loved ones.

Trend line. The line created by plotting blood sugar levels as points on a chart with time along the bottom axis traveling from left to right and the level of glucose (sugar) displayed on the up and down axis from lowest (at the bottom) to higher (at the top). Trend lines can be viewed by the CGM user along different periods of time to get different views about how slowly or quickly BG trends are changing.

Tunneling. The passage of unabsorbed insulin around the outside of a pump catheter upward along the length of the catheter towards the surface of the skin. Tunneling is a cause for higher blood sugars due to lack of proper insulin delivery. In more severe cases that go undetected, diabetic ketoacidosis can happen. Most catheter sites tunnel after they've been inserted several days and if there has been some pulling on the site itself. This tugging may serve to dislodge the seal between the skin and the catheter itself.

Type 1 diabetes. Type 1 diabetes (formerly called juvenile-onset or insulin-dependent) is most often caused by losing the ability to make the hormone insulin. Without enough insulin in the body, the cells are not able to take in enough sugar for their energy needs. In some cases, the body will start to break down fat as a backup source of energy. When this goes to an extreme, a problem called diabetic ketoacidosis (DKA) happens, which can be deadly.

Waiting for the Bend. A core Sugar Surfing principle. Watching the CGM trend line for a change in the shape of the line. This suggests a change in the blood sugar levels is happening either from insulin, food, exercise, stress or even some medicines. Waiting for the bend describes a valuable Sugar Surfing method to better time food intake several minutes after taking the corresponding dose of insulin.

Wet shot. When liquid (mixed with or without a small amount of blood) is seen at the site of an insulin injection, the presumption is that some of the insulin was not delivered. The amount of insulin lost in a wet shot is nearly impossible to judge. Therefore most persons will make a note of this and watch BG trends or levels more carefully to determine what effect (if any) the wet shot had on the BG levels. It is generally not a good idea to attempt a second injection with the intent of making up for the lost insulin. Simply monitor blood sugar and use Sugar Surfing techniques to keep blood sugar in your desired range.

Wipeout. A Sugar Surfing term borrowed from the ocean surfing term to experience a sudden loss of "in the moment" blood sugar control. This can mean an extremely high or low blood sugar result after being relatively successful in your Sugar Surfing efforts. Wipeouts happen and can be managed and even prevented. But even when they happen, they should not discourage you from your Sugar Surfing efforts. Rather, use them to learn valuable lessons from what happened and improve on your next attempt.

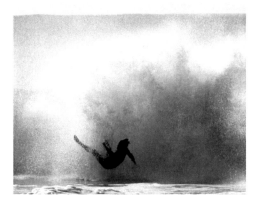

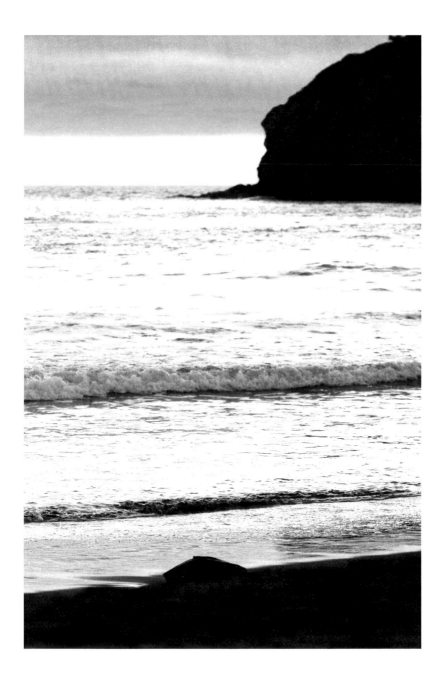

About My Co-Author

Kevin McMahon began his work in diabetes in 2001 after his daughter, Darby, was diagnosed with type 1 diabetes. With a technology background in computers, mobile networks and emerging smart phones, advancing diabetes technology was only a matter of time. By 2002 his team was in the field with the first automated and real-time remote blood sugar monitoring /communication solution anywhere in the world. This was followed up by several additional tools including a service for patients to receive computer generated personalized diabetes education immediately following their blood sugar checks.

In 2003, his original design of the Remotely Monitored Artificial Pancreas was submitted to JDRF, the US Army and the NIH for grant consideration. Since then, McMahon and his collaborators, including myself, developed many innovative tools for use by patients and clinicians designed to simplify daily tasks while simultaneously educating patients and their caregivers. Beyond just the technology, his research is still influencing how companies design diabetes products that we all use each and every day.

Integrating all of the available technologies and helping to discover new ones represents an important dimension toward realizing practical and safe step-wise advancements along the road to an artificial pancreas. In addition to the many hours spent in support of Sugar Surfing, Mr. McMahon is an advisor to several startup companies within the field of advanced medical device and information technology systems. Kevin also regularly contributes to articles published in respected medical journals.

His inspiration comes from his daughters, Mackenzie and Darby, and his very supportive family. He lives in the San Francisco Bay Area.

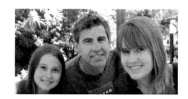